Effective Coaching in Healthcare

Ruth Hadikin BSc(Hons) Cert Ed ADM RM RN
Professional Life Coach, specialising in personal and business transformation

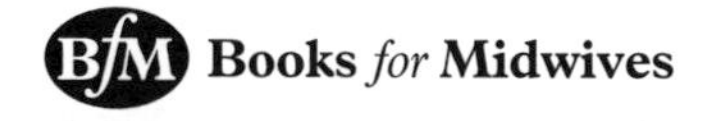

EDINBURGH LONDON NEW YORK OXFORD PHILADELPHIA ST LOUIS
SYDNEY TORONTO 2004

ISBN 0 7506 5498 8

British Library Cataloguing in Publication Data
A catalogue record for this book is available from the British Library

Library of Congress Cataloging in Publication Data
A catalog record for this book is available from the Library of Congress

Medical knowledge is constantly changing. Standard safety precautions must be followed, but as new research and clinical experience broaden our knowledge, changes in treatment and drug therapy may become necessary or appropriate. Readers are advised to check the most current product information provided by the manufacturer of each drug to be administered to verify the recommended dose, the method and duration of administration, and contraindications. It is the responsibility of the practitioner, relying on experience and knowledge of the patient, to determine dosages and the best treatment for each individual patient. Neither the Publisher nor the author assumes any liability for any injury and/or damage to persons or property arising from this publication.

The Publisher

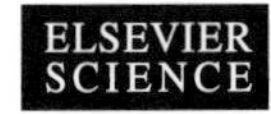

your source for books, journals and multimedia in the health sciences

www.elsevierhealth.com

The publisher's policy is to use **paper manufactured from sustainable forests**

Printed in China

Effective Coaching in Healthcare

For Books for Midwives:

Commissioning Editor: Mary Seager
Project Editor: Catharine Steers
Project Manager: Morven Dean
Design: George Ajayi

Contents

About the author

Previously a community midwife and midwife teacher, Ruth Hadikin BSc(Hons) Cert Ed ADM RM RN is a business and life coach specialising in emotional intelligence, stress management and personal, professional and organisational development. She has published many articles and co-authored *The Bullying Culture* with Muriel O'Driscoll. With appearances on BBC television and radio, Ruth is a popular speaker who offers workshops, teleclasses, international coaching by phone or e-mail, personal and group coaching on living your best life. Ruth is founder and director of Ruth Hadikin Associates: coaching, development and training, based in Lancashire.

You are invited to try a taste of coaching for yourself. To schedule a free introductory 30-minute coaching session over the telephone, or invite Ruth to speak to your professional group or association, contact her by phone or e-mail.

Tel: 01704 896039
e-mail: ruth@dreamcoach.co.uk
website: www.dreamcoach.co.uk

Forewords

Dame Lorna Muirhead
President of the Royal College of Midwives

Over the last two decades there has been a radical shift in the way people have been expected to work. For most of us employed in the NHS today, unprecedented stresses and strains are becoming a part of everyday life, as we seek to provide a service on which the public places increasing demands, and for which successive governments have made inadequate provision.

Many people feel overworked, stressed and undervalued. Perhaps above all, they feel unable to change the situation, or to influence undesirable cultures which have become part of everyday working life.

Medicine and technology are advancing at an exciting and rapid pace. Whilst this continual development brings benefits to many, it nevertheless makes the workplace an area of endless change, which compounds the difficulties experienced by an already stretched workforce.

Domestic life, too, has changed almost beyond recognition even from our parents' day, and many now find themselves pursuing a career, keeping up to date professionally, running a home, and caring for children or other dependent relatives. Is it any wonder, then, that many of us get to a point where we need to do 'something about our lives'? What, we ask ourselves, can we do to address the things we meet daily, with which we are coping badly? How can we get out of the undesirable rut in which we have become stuck? Is there anything we ourselves can do to change the effects of a negative or harmful culture, where it exists in our professional or domestic life? Waiting for others to change things for us often proves unrealistic.

Modern problems need modern solutions, and this book about life coaching offers that modern approach. With its help you will begin to raise your own awareness of how *you* can change those aspects of your life which you feel are unsatisfactory. The book will steer you to make major or minor adjustments to your behaviour or way of thinking, actions which will help you to take greater control of your life and rid you of as many negative influences as possible. You, in turn, could become the catalyst to assist your colleagues. Imagine the transformation of the workplace where people have actually learned to cope better with all they are expected to do.

Not only can coaching change individuals, it is available and successful in groups. Trusts and other workplaces can only benefit from a workforce revitalised through successful coaching.

Like its author, the book is full of common sense, harnessed to knowledge and a sincere desire to help those who need it.

Ishbel Kargar
Retired Secretary, The Association of Radical Midwives

From time to time, ideas emerge which seem to be in tune with current needs, and this book falls into that category. There is much talk lately about the need for personal development and awareness of one's potential, though the means to achieve these aims are not universally available. In this book, Ruth Hadikin has provided an excellent pathway which, if taken, will enable healthcare workers to improve their own self-awareness, attain personal goals, and also contribute to a major culture change: towards a more enlightened, sympathetic treatment of the people working within healthcare and of those using the service.

Fortunately, programmes such as the coaching which Ruth Hadikin describes in this book can help individuals to overcome obstacles to their own professional and personal development, and to gain self-confidence, enabling them to recognise where changes should be made, not only in their own lives, but within the organisation in which they work. They then realise that there are far better ways of making an organisation run efficiently than the hierarchical system which ignores personal feelings and aspirations. It is human nature to want to please those we respect, and such respect does not come from being made to feel inadequate, inferior and useless.

Enlightened managers have long realised that the organisation will thrive when the workers are valued, not only in terms of financial reward, but also in terms of expressed appreciation and encouragement for the quality of the work done. Those who work in such organisations communicate their job satisfaction to others outside the organisation, and it is no surprise that job vacancies are easily filled by such a company.

Many people have feelings of dissatisfaction with their chosen way of life, perhaps resenting the lack of job satisfaction, but it is often difficult to pin-point the reasons for such feelings, and even less easy to see a way to remedy the situation. Ruth's book shows a way out. Her message is that coaching can be a dynamic tool to bring about a beneficial change in one's outlook, enabling one to move on to a more rewarding way of life, and to contribute more actively to beneficial changes within the workplace and at home.

Ruth gives many very useful examples of the value of coaching, starting with the process of recognising how to resolve a difficult personal situation. However, the concept of coaching has a wider remit, with regard to a gradual elimination of the culture of bullying. Coaching works on the basis that any organisation, whether a small group of people, or a huge one such as the NHS, consists of individuals, and those individuals need to value and respect each other for the organisation to survive and prosper. It is an idea which has come into its time.

Acknowledgements

In keeping with the spirit of coaching, I would like to acknowledge everyone who has acknowledged, nurtured, inspired, motivated, enabled, empowered and supported me to make this book possible. None of us ever does anything alone. The following is a list of all those who have provided support, coaching, a role model, inspiration, encouragement, a listening ear, a kind word, constructive feedback, resources, websites, references, journal articles, their time, their energy, proof-reading and much, much more. This book has been a team effort.

There are many, many more people who will never know how much they helped by just offering a little encouragement, or a kind word at the right moment. Even those I have never met have contributed by generously giving of themselves and sharing their inspirational work. I am grateful to each one for having the courage to be who they are.

I encourage you to begin to acknowledge all those who have helped you to become who you are today.

Dr Ron Arndt
Eunice Brookes
Harry Brookes
Henrietta Brookes
Robert Brookes
Tania Berlow
Bernie Boyle
Don Boyle
Jane Brendgen
Kimberly Bryant
Julia Cameron
Dr Margaret Collins
Brenda Cowley
Lama Surya Das
Barbara Deakin
Coen DeGroot
Bridgit Dimond
Rachelle Disbennett-Lee
Clare Dobson
Elizabeth Ferguson
Donna Fisher
Mahatma Ghandi
Barbara Gibson
Daniel Goleman
Dominic Goulding
Gill Goulding

Suzy Greaves
Soleira Green
Andrea Grieveson
Andrew Hadikin
Glenn Hadikin
Jamie Hadikin
Kay Hadikin
Paddy Hadikin
Stephen Hadikin
Nicola Hall
Francena Hancock
Louise Hay
Anne Hayes
Nikki Hennessy
Fran Henry
Anne Heron
Laura Hess
Barbara Marx Hubbard
Sue Jamieson
Ishbel Kargar
Byron Katie
Dianna Keel
Dr Susan Kersley
Clare Lambe
Julie Lambert
Liam Lathum
Jackie Lathum
Thomas Leonard
Harriet Lerner
Arlene Mann
Linda Markley
Abraham Maslow
Theresa McGouran
Alison Moss
Lorna Muirhead DBE
John Nagy
Muriel O'Driscoll
Sheila O'Sullivan
Brenda Peacock
M Scott Peck
Jay Perry
Chris Pyke
Lorna Ramsay
James Redfield
Don Miguel Riuz
Anthony Robbins
Clare Robson
Carl Rogers
Anna Rushton
Mary Seager
Bernie Sharkey
Mark Slaski
Dr John Stephenson
Susan Swithin
Dr Kem Thompson
Jacqui Tillyard
Zoran Tordorovich
Sandy Tremp
Scott Tremp
Sandy Vilas
Louise Waller
Neil Donald Walsch
Fiona Watson
Dr Robin Whittemore
Laura Whitworth
Oprah Winfrey
David Woodward
Lynda Woodward
Myra Wylupek
Gary Zukav

Introduction

Our creative dreams and yearnings come from a divine source.
As we move toward our dreams we move toward our divinity.

Julia Cameron, *The Artist's Way*

This book is unlike many healthcare texts that you may have read before. This book takes us on a journey of self-discovery. As you would expect, it introduces the topic of coaching, including an introduction to life coaching. It summarises what coaching entails, with various coaching definitions, coaching models and a theory of why coaching is emerging as a distinct profession at this moment in time. In addition to this theoretical base, it is hoped that this book will provide you with an experience of coaching.

This is a book about change yet, paradoxically, it is more about how making subtle changes in you can affect your family, organisation and the world around you. As you will see as you read on, coaching is about a relationship between the coach and the coachee. For our purposes here, let us say that you are the coachee and I am your coach. Although reading a book can never substitute for a 'live' coaching relationship, it is my ambitious goal to give you some experience of coaching through reading this book. I hope that you will begin to be an observer of yourself. I hope that you will pause and do the suggested exercises, rather than just glossing over them to read the next bit. It is my hope that in reading this book you will begin a journey that will ultimately bring you home to your Self.

In keeping with the spirit of coaching, I have written in a familiar, personalised style and have set fieldwork exercises at key points throughout the book. I have also written in the feminine. This is in honour of the fact that the majority of healthcare providers are indeed women, and for ease of reading and writing. The term 'client' equally applies to coachees in private practice and clients of the health service. The term 'coachee' applies to anyone being coached, including those who are employees and are coached by their manager. To avoid confusion, the term 'coachee' has been used throughout the book to denote the person being coached. The term 'client' refers to clients of healthcare.

Coaching, as a tool to accelerate personal and business development, is currently taking the business and management world by storm. Its contribution to phenomenal transformation at organisational and personal levels has resulted in coaching being widely adopted in other disciplines.

As with facilitation and nurturing, coaching does not directly achieve anything in and of itself. It is not a cause and effect concept. Coaching creates an environment in which development and growth can take place. Coaches are like gardeners who have an interactive relationship with their plants. The gardener focuses all her attention on creating the optimum conditions for growth, and then it is up to the plants to 'do' the growing. Similarly, in coaching the results cannot be guaranteed any more than they can in gardening. Like the gardener, the coach can create the perfect environment for growth and be 80% certain that, barring natural disasters and circumstances beyond our control which could devastate the crop, the crop will flourish.

It is my intention that this book provides an understanding of the coaching philosophy, the psychology of coaching, the skills involved and the many applications of coaching. It is also my hope that coaching can be viewed as both a method of achieving culture change within healthcare and as a potential part of the culture itself.

Culture is defined by sociologists as:

The values, beliefs, customs, rules and regulations of a group or society.

(Haralambos, 1986)

The culture in the health service has become pretty toxic over the years. Working in the health service could be detrimental to your own health, especially your psychological and emotional health, if not eventually your physical and spiritual health. The term 'psychotoxic' has been used to describe these psychologically damaging conditions. In *The Bullying Culture* (Hadikin and O'Driscoll, 2000) Muriel O'Driscoll and I identified the psychotoxic culture that permeates the national health service (NHS). Where bullying is the problem, coaching is the solution. Yet it is much more than a solution to only one problem. Bullying is a negative interaction or a series of negative interactions forming a negative relationship. Coaching is an effective antidote to bullying. As you will see, coaching offers a way to convert this psychotoxic environment into a nurturing, healthy environment. It does this by focusing on how to stop negativity and replace it with positive, rewarding, affirming interactions which lead to positive healthy relationships. This change, which takes place on a personal level, has far-reaching implications throughout our family, the NHS and society.

The concept of emotional intelligence or EQ runs throughout this book. Emotional intelligence is a term used to describe an emotional maturity and our ability to not only use emotional information but to integrate it with our thoughts and actions (Slaski, 2002). Coaching facilitates a process of healing, growth and development whereby we raise our EQ.

A central tenet of the coaching philosophy is defining a clear sense of self. This is important, because coaching is about real people, living real lives, with real dreams, overcoming real obstacles. It is not about some hypothetical other 'one'. It is about your Self and my Self. Our Selves. Coaching is about helping ordinary people to meet extraordinary challenges in their lives, by being clear about who they really are: unique individuals with unique gifts, talents and strengths. A unique sense of Self. I have never met a talentless person, though I meet many who have never discovered what their real strengths are. They have never discovered a true sense of Self. Hopefully this book will inspire you to discover yours, and go on to inspire others to discover theirs.

I request that you do the exercises in this book. In coaching, you are responsible for yourself. You therefore always have a choice: do all of it, do some of it, or say 'no'. However, if you say 'no', what will you do instead? Commit to some action to further your own goals. My aim in writing this book is for you to both feel that you have been coached a little, and to feel that you could apply coaching skills in your practice. A tall order, especially when coaching is experiential by nature and you are reading a book which is, at best, theoretical.

I also request that, if you don't do so already, you begin to keep a journal. Not just an ordinary journal – a coaching journal. I don't want it to be a report of your daily activity: '6am: got up, ate breakfast, drove to work', etc. Your coaching journal is where you record your observations of your Self. As you read on you will discover the importance of being an objective observer of self (Chapter 2). For example:

How do you feel?

Are you anxious?

Or is it anger?

What presses your buttons?

Do you react or respond?

Begin observing YOU. By the end of this book, hopefully, you will be an excellent observer of yourself. You may also have become the best expert on you. This book could help you to discover that for yourself, and then believe that your clients are also the best experts on themselves. This could change your whole approach to the way you run your practice. You may, if you choose, decide to become a coach practitioner. This may simply mean that you adopt a coaching style in your interactions with your clients and colleagues, or indeed you may choose to set up structured coaching sessions.

This is a textbook with a difference. It is my intention that it changes your life in some way, however small. It is difficult within a text to convey the experience of a process. At best, all we may end up with is a description of the theory of the process. However, that will not deter me from attempting to give you as much experience of the process of coaching as I can possibly muster within these pages. Even so, despite all my best intentions to coach, in requesting you begin a journal and giving you exercises to take action upon and reflect, it is still not possible to experience coaching by reading a book. Coaching is an active process, and trying to experience coaching by reading about it is like trying to learn to drive by sitting in a classroom and reading a driving manual. Sooner or later, if you're going to be a driver, you have to get into the car. To compensate for this deficiency, I have covered many of the topics of personal growth that would come up over a series of coaching calls with my clients. If I appear to digress from the topic of 'coaching in healthcare' you will find that it will be into the area of developing you, as you read. So pay attention, and be open and willing to be coached. In our short journey together through this book, during those times where we appear to digress completely from the theory of coaching in healthcare, we may very well be in the process of coaching YOU!

If this book inspires you to explore coaching further, I invite you to choose a coach for yourself. Use the coach directory at the back of this book to create a shortlist of the six coaches that appeal to you most. Call each one and speak with them about how they would coach you. In this way you will experience different coaching styles and approaches. Since coaching is, at the moment, an unregulated profession you may wish to ask about each coach's training and experience, in addition to their fees, before you hire yourself a coach. You will then be in a position to jump into the water and try personal coaching for yourself.

My vision for the future of healthcare is that every practitioner has a personal coach of their own choosing and that peer coaching becomes established throughout the NHS. This would foster a positive, supportive working environment in which NHS employees at every level are nurtured, acknowledged and encouraged to develop their potential. If this seems impossible, too expensive or too far-fetched, let me show you how it can be done. Read on.

1

What is coaching?

A good coach will make his players see what they can be rather than what they are.

Ara Parasheghian

Coaching is a new profession which has evolved in the field of personal development. Though sports coaches have been around for quite some time, personal coaching is a new profession which has arisen out of business consultancy. Management consultants, businesses and organisations began to realise, as did sports coaches before them, that coaching was more effective than consulting or 'advising'. The reason is simple: people are more effective when they take responsibility and are accountable for their own actions. In a sense, coaching is nothing new. There have been coaches throughout recorded history, though 'coaching' may not be the term that was used to describe what they did.

DEFINITIONS OF COACHING

There is no universal definition of what coaching is. I have always said that coaching is simply helping others to realise their potential. However, I also love the idea of liberating human potential. I was once told a story about working elephants in Sri Lanka who, upon 'retirement' from their labour, had their shackles removed only to stay in the same place where they had stood for decades. Why don't they run away? Simply because they have no experience of anything else. They know of no other way to be. I think that people are the same. We develop a routine, stick with it, and even if someone asks us or invites us to change, we don't know how, or to what. To what would we change? What could we become? We need to experience another way of being, even if only a vision, before we can become it. We need to know that there is something more over the horizon, something worth having, something that is possible, and have a plan of how to get there. It is not enough to be free, we have to *know* that we are free, and know how to live freely. This means recognising where we have choices. Coaching was the process that both enabled me to recognise where I had choices in life that I never knew I had, and invited me to explore my own horizons. So I would like to offer a definition of coaching as 'liberating human potential'.

It might also help us to understand the nature of coaching by exploring some contemporary definitions of coaching. The Coaches Training Institute define coaching as:

> *a powerful alliance designed to forward and enhance the lifelong process of human learning, effectiveness and fulfillment.*
>
> *(The Coaches Training Institute, 2002)*

This definition is helpful in that it includes the 'alliance' aspect of the coaching relationship. For personal coaching to be effective, the relationship is important. Coaching involves a partnership between coachee and coach. The coach is regarded as a peer rather than an expert, authority or senior. This definition refers to what the authors term the 'co-active' coaching model (see further in this chapter for discussion of this model), again emphasising the equality of status, partnership, and equality of personal responsibility within the coaching relationship. This creates a conducive environment in which synergy takes place. Synergy is a term used to describe the effect created by two or more people, whereby the result is greater than the sum of the two parts. The Oxford English Dictionary defines synergy as:

> *the combined effect... that exceeds the sum of their individual effects* [and] *increased effectiveness or achievement produced by combined action or cooperation*
>
> *(Pearsall and Trumble, 1996)*

Some organisations distinguish between facilitation and coaching, whilst others view facilitation as an aspect of coaching. For example, The School of Coaching at The Industrial Society defines coaching as:

The art of facilitating the performance, learning and development of another

whereas the popular US coach training company 'CoachU' makes the following distinction between group coaching and facilitation:

Coaching is focused on the person (who), whereas facilitation is often focused on the process (how). A Coach usually gives more input and direction than a facilitator, and makes specific requests of the participants. A Coach usually asks more of the group than a facilitator does (e.g. to produce more)

(CoachU, 1999)

Coaching is a process which focuses on the person. It might even be more accurate to think of coaching as a process which facilitates the development of the 'self'. Carl Rogers (1961) suggested that the process of becoming a person, or our 'selves', is part of a 'maturation' process which is either latent or evident in all individuals.

The individual has within himself the capacity and the tendency, latent if not evident, to move forward toward maturity. In a suitable psychological climate this tendency is released, and becomes actual rather than potential.

(Rogers, 1961)

Effective coaching creates such a 'suitable psychological climate' in which the positive, empowering, encouraging and supportive environment promotes growth, and potential becomes realised. This environment has to be felt as real, rather than illusory, for it to be beneficial. It is therefore essential that the coach is sincere and genuine in her desire to move the coachee forward. The coach must genuinely want the coachee to realise her potential.

The contrast between contemporary definitions of personal coaching, and the traditional view of coaching, can be seen in this definition of the verb 'to coach', taken from the 1996 edition of The Oxford English Dictionary:

a. to train or teach (a pupil, sports team etc.) as a coach

b. give hints to; prime with facts

In the same edition 'A Coach' is defined as simply:

a. an instructor or trainer in sport.

b. a private tutor

(Pearsall and Trumble, 1996)

This contrast illustrates how coaching, as a profession in its own right, is evolving away from the traditional view of coaching where 'the coach' was viewed as the expert in a particular subject and 'coaching' implied imparting knowledge or, as described above, priming with facts.

In the contemporary view, personal coaches need not have any knowledge of the coachee's area of expertise; they are considered experts in the process of coaching itself. This is not to say that coaches do not have areas of expertise, which they do, but that it is not necessary for the coach to draw upon such expertise for coaching to be effective.

This is an unusual concept, which makes little sense if we take a traditional view of coaching. How, for example, could a Football Coach coach a team and yet know nothing about football? Yet today you may have a business coach who knows little, if anything, about her coachee's business. This is because, rather than being an expert in the coachee's field, it is the coach's role to be an 'expert' in the process of coaching. It is her role to possess the skill and art of enabling the coachee to become the expert in her own field.

The International Coach Federation (ICF) exists as a body to set standards and ethics for this newly-emerging profession (see Figures 1.1 and 1.2). In their document 'The Nature and Scope of Coaching' (see Figure 1.2) they state:

Coaches are experts in the coaching process and may not have specific knowledge of a given subject area or industry. Where coaches have expertise in other areas, they may use it to facilitate the coaching process.

(ICF, 2002)

I recently coached a young man whose stated goal was to race a BOSS F1. He had written this on a postcard which I had given out at a talk, upon which I requested people write their life goal. I looked at his card, blinked, and looked again. I assumed 'F1' must refer to Formula One motor racing; however, I had thought, being familiar with Liverpudlian vernacular, that perhaps what he meant by a 'boss' F1 was a good one! I was wrong, of course. Those of you who are familiar with motor racing will know that a

The Nature and Scope of Coaching

Part One: With Respect to Psychotherapy
Definition: In all of the following statements, the word 'client' is used to denote the person who is being coached, regardless of who is paying for the service.

WHO THE CLIENT IS
The individual coaching client is someone who wants to reach one or more of the following: a higher level of performance, learning, or satisfaction. The client is not seeking emotional healing or relief from psychological pain.

The coaching client can take action to move towards a goal with the support of the coach. The successful client is not excessively limited in the ability to take action or overly hesitant to make this kind of progress.

HOW SERVICE IS DELIVERED
Coaches and clients arrange the schedule and means of contact (e.g., in person, by phone, or via e-mail) that serve them both. They are not constrained to follow a standardized schedule or means of contact.

THE RELATIONSHIP IN COACHING
A coach relates to the client as a partner. A coach does not relate to the client from a position of an expert, authority, or healer.

Coach and client together choose the focus, format, and desired outcomes for their work. The client does not relinquish the responsibility for creating and maintaining these nor does the coach take full responsibility for them.

RESULTS
Coaching is designed to help clients improve their learning and performance, and enhance their quality of life. Coaching does not focus directly on relieving psychological pain or treating cognitive or emotional disorders.

TIME FRAMES
Coaching concentrates primarily on the present and future. Coaching does not focus on the past or on the past's impact on the present.

Coaching uses information from the client's past to clarify where the client is today. It does not depend on resolution of the past to move the client forward.

EMOTIONS
Coaching assumes the presence of emotional reactions to life events and that clients are capable of expressing and handling their emotions. Coaching is not psychotherapy and emotional healing is not the focus of coaching.

RELATIONSHIP TO PSYCHOTHERAPY
Coaching can be used concurrently with psychotherapeutic work. It is not used as a substitute for psychotherapeutic work.

ADVICE
Advice, opinions, or suggestions are occasionally offered in coaching. Both parties understand that the client is free to accept or decline what is offered and takes the ultimate responsibility for action. The coach is not discouraged from offering advice, opinions or suggestions on occasion.

REQUESTING
A coach makes a request of the client to promote action toward the client's desired outcome. A coach does not make such a request in order to fix the client's problem or understand the client's past.

Figure 1.1 The nature and scope of coaching. Part one: with respect to psychotherapy (Reproduced, with permission, from the International Coach Federation, 2002)

The Nature and Scope of Coaching

Part II: With Respect to Consulting
Definition: In all of the following statements, the word 'client' is used to denote the person who is being coached, regardless of who is paying for the service.

EXPERTISE
Coaches are experts in the coaching process and may not have specific knowledge of a given subject area or industry. Where coaches have expertise in other areas, they may use it to facilitate the coaching process. Coaches do not use this particular expertise to diagnose, direct, or design solutions for the client.

RELATIONSHIP
Relationship is the foundation of coaching. The coach and client intentionally develop a relationship which is characterized by a growing and mutual appreciation and respect for each other as individuals. This relationship is not an adjunct to or byproduct of the coaching. Nor is it based on the client's position or performance.

USE OF INFORMATION
In coaching, information drawn from the client is used by the coach to promote the client's awareness and choice of action. This information is not used to evaluate performance or produce reports for anyone but the person being coached.

SCOPE
Coaching has the freedom and flexibility to address a wide variety of personal and professional topics. In any given coaching relationship, coach and client alone determine the scope of their work. Coaching is not necessarily restricted to a narrowly defined issue not is its scope determined in any other way.

CONTRIBUTION TO RESULTS
In coaching, any contribution the coach makes to producing the client's desired outcome is through ongoing interaction wth the client. The coach's role does not include producing a contracted product or result outside of the coaching sessions.

ONGOING IMPACT
Coaching is designed to provide clients with a greater capacity to produce results and a greater confidence in their ability to do so. It is intended that clients do not leave coaching with a perception that they need to rely on a coach in order to produce similar results in the future.

Figure 1.2 The nature and scope of coaching. Part two: with respect to consulting (Reproduced, with permission, from the International Coach Federation, 2002)

BOSS F1 is actually a make of Formula One motor. The point is though, that my ignorance of Formula One racing actually made me a better coach for him. It removed any temptation on my part to attempt to be the 'expert' on the subject and left me free to coach from pure curiosity and my interest in him as the coachee.

My questions, therefore, ran along the lines of:

How did you get into Formula One?

What turns you on about F1?

What experience have you had?

How do people get into it as a profession?

How many other F1 drivers do you know?

What circles do they mix in?

How can you get to meet them?

What have you tried already?

What do you need to do next?

Obviously I didn't just 'fire' my questions at him one after the other like this; I waited for his answers, listened, and allowed the process of coaching to unfold. This is where the 'magic' of coaching happens. In telling me, he realised he knew more about the subject than he thought he did, or indeed gave himself credit for. He realised he was much nearer his goal than he imagined, he was on his way and could recognise how far he had already come. He could identify more steps along the way. He became clear about what he needed to do next, and what kind of timeframe to put around it. He gained the confidence and motivation to take the necessary action and agreed to do some of it that very week. He made a commitment to himself to take action steps, and gave me a deadline by which he would feedback to me with the results.

This illustrates some of the key concepts of coaching which I will be discussing in more detail later in this book. Into the coaching relationship, the coach brings skills and qualities such as questioning, curiosity, intuition and listening. The coachee brings commitment, action and accountability. The synergy in the relationship produces clarity, inspiration and focus for the coachee. Clarity and focus are often cited as top reasons why people hire a coach.

Intuition? Yes, you may not have noticed intuition in the above example, but it was there. In coaching, the 'hunch', 'gut feeling', 'inkling' or 'intuition' is acknowledged as an essential part of the process. More often than not, we will find that we ask the most appropriate question of a client when we have simply had nothing more than an inexplicable urge to do so. Denying the client the benefit of our intuition is to deprive them of a valuable tool, a valuable insight into their situation. It is wise to let the client know that it is our intuition that we are drawing upon, and to ask their permission to share our hunch.

The International Coach Federation offers the following definition of coaching:

Professional coaches provide an ongoing partnership designed to help clients produce fulfilling results in their personal and professional lives. Coaches help people improve their performances and enhance the quality of their lives.

Coaches are trained to listen, to observe and to customize their approach to individual client needs. They seek to elicit solutions and strategies from the client; they believe the client is naturally creative and resourceful. The coach's job is to provide support to enhance the skills, resources, and creativity that the client already has.

(ICF, 2002)

Coaching focuses, in part, on taking action that moves us forward or helps us develop. The request for action is a fundamental part of each coaching session. In taking the action that has been requested of her, the coachee stretches herself, is challenged and often tries things she has never done before. We can see how it is not necessary for the coach even to know how to do whatever it is that the coachee wants to do. Our clients, colleagues and coachees need not be limited by our limitations.

Good coaching, and good mentoring for that matter, can and should take a performer beyond the limitations of the coach or mentor's own knowledge.

(Whitmore, 1996, p.11.)

Another face of contemporary coaching is that of the Life Coach. I choose this term to describe what I do, because it encompasses life situations. I coach around life skills; I coach around relationships both at home and at work; I coach around emotional intelligence; I coach around career transition; I coach around personal change and I coach around spirituality, to name but a few. These are coaching situations. My coaching style is to adopt a client-centred approach. My coaching is client-led and 'holistic' or whole-person coaching. This means the coaching session is led by whatever challenges the client is facing in the present moment and I always work with the client's agenda. The kind of coaching I do, based on the search for self, encompasses everything and anything that life throws our way.

One of my favourite definitions of a Life Coach comes from fellow coach Carole Gaskell:

[a life coach is...] someone who inspires and supports you to live your best life, doing what you enjoy.

Carole Gaskell, founder and Managing Director of The Lifecoaching Company (www.lifecoaching-company.co.uk)

COACHING PHILOSOPHY

The philosophy underpinning personal coaching is that the coachee is creative, resourceful and whole. The coachee has the answers within herself and it is the coach's job to help her to realise that. Coaching is based on a health model rather than a sickness model. The coachee is whole, complete and capable of resolving her own challenges. The coach becomes a partner with the coachee in achieving her goals.

Coaching offers a non-therapeutic resource for people who are undergoing the process of transition, i.e. people who are in the process of becoming something: becoming a nurse or midwife, becoming a leader, becoming a manager, becoming a mother, becoming ourselves. In a sense we are all becoming something. We are undergoing a personal transformation that will see us change from the metaphorical caterpillar into a butterfly. Staying the same is not an option. Individually we experience a process of living, learning and maturing. As a species we are evolving. It is the nature of evolution to gravitate towards our successes, to be motivated to be our best. We are becoming better versions of who we can be, reaching our potential. We are in the process of what Maslow (1982) described as self-actualisation (see Psychology of Self, Chapter 2). We are innately attracted towards self-actualisation.

As we are attracted to whatever appeals to us in order to continue our personal growth, we experience a dilemma between what we feel we want to do, how we feel we want to act or behave, and what 'society', our peers, our parents, family, friends, wider society tells us we 'should', 'ought' or 'must' do. Whatever is 'normal', or more accurately 'typical', for 'someone like us'. This gives us a feeling of being different, being 'wrong' in some way. It also means that we allow others to define who 'someone like us' is or should be. Others define who we are, and we find it difficult to keep to an externally-defined role. How difficult is it to continually live up to someone else's expectation of what a 'good' nurse or midwife 'should' be? Far better to set your own standard and be the best midwife or nurse that you know how to be.

Toward Trust of Self

Still another way of describing this pattern which I see in each client is to say that increasingly he [sic] trusts and values the process which is himself. Watching my clients, I have come to a much better understanding of creative people. El Greco, for example, must have realised as he looked at some of his early work, that 'good artists do not paint like that'. But somehow he trusted his own experiencing of life, the process of himself, sufficiently that he could go on expressing his own unique perceptions. It was as though he could say, 'Good artists do not paint like this, but I paint like this.' Or to move to another field, Ernest Hemingway was surely aware that 'good writers do not write like this'. But fortunately he moved toward being Hemingway, being himself, rather than toward someone else's conception of a good writer. Einstein seems to have been unusually oblivious to the fact that good physicists did not think his kind of thoughts. Rather than drawing back because of his inadequate academic preparation in physics, he simply moved toward being Einstein, toward thinking his own thoughts, toward being as truly and deeply himself as he could. This is not a phenomenon which occurs only in the artist or the genius. Time and again in my clients, I have seen simple people become significant and creative in their own spheres, as they have developed more trust of the processes going on within themselves, and have dared to feel their own feelings, live by values which they discover within, and express themselves in their own unique ways.

(Rogers, 1961)

We are torn between our need to belong to our group (family, peers, organisation) and our need to have a definition of ourselves as unique, distinct and different from others.

A journey to authenticity: our search for Self

What makes one person draw back when they feel inadequate, whilst another, like Einstein, seems to be confident that being himself is enough? There are many psychological theories, some of which will be discussed in greater detail in Chapter 2. What is important for us as coaches to know is that, like Einstein, Hemingway and El Greco, we are all capable of becoming more of our true selves. There is growing evidence that we can measure and improve our emotional intelligence or EQ (Salovey and Mayer, 1990; Goleman, 1996; Slaski and Cartwright, 2002). This suggests that temperament, once thought to be fixed at birth, can change, evolve and grow with us as we mature through life. More importantly, we can exercise choice in the matter. We can make choices which honour our sense of Self and bring us more into alignment with who we want to be, rather than our externally prescribed role. As we are exposed to different experiences, we adapt to our environment. We are literally evolving in our own lifetimes. (See emotional intelligence in Chapter 2.)

A personal life coach is someone who can be with you through this process. A sort of 'life midwife'. A coaching client, after six months in post in a new and challenging role, said: 'I feel as if I have birthed this role, and you have been my 'midwife' throughout the process!'

What did she mean? In this new role there were no precedents, and nobody to tell her what she should be doing. Her manager confided that she did not understand the role and was waiting for my client to show her. She had to put her own mark on the role and create the blueprint for future generations.

What did she mean when she said that she had 'birthed' the process? She had come into a new role, completely in the dark, much as an expectant mother does. Something big was happening and she was in the middle of it, but she didn't know exactly how it was going to work out, nor what, specifically, she was supposed to DO. She went through a process of self-discovery. She asked herself:

What are my strengths, skills and talents?

How can I best apply them to create this new role?

What are the new skills that I will need to acquire?

Specifically, which interpersonal skills, communication skills, management skills and leadership skills do I have already, and which will I need to learn?

With prompting from her coach, and in answering these questions, she took herself through a process of self-inquiry. It was very much a creative process and in order to reach her potential she needed to re-connect with her creativity. In a sense it was a process of evolution. She was at the cutting edge of personal and professional (human!) evolution and was personally evolving into a new kind of leader for the future. She was on a journey of personal self-discovery as she inquired 'who am I, in this role?' She developed a strong sense of Self. She became defined by her values rather than by her role. She became authentic and felt as though she was more of her 'true' Self.

So what was my role as the 'midwife', the coach, in this 'birthing' process? Imagine a space in your busy week where the focus is entirely on you, and where you are in a relationship with a professional whose only goal is to move you forward to reach your potential by holding you accountable to you. A professional who listens, and really hears you. A professional whose job is to listen 100% to you, then feedback what they hear you saying you want. Then holds you to it – unless you don't really want it, of course!. A professional whose responsibility is to help you to be responsible to you. Even if this means telling you the truth when it sometimes hurts. A professional who will tell you exactly where you are sabotaging yourself and show you another way to be, rather than your settling for being less than who you are and can be. A professional who listens without judgement, so you can drop any pretence or social mask and simply be who you really are. A professional who has empathy and compassion but doesn't let you off the hook. Someone who cares about you, is curious about you and is committed to you and your growth. Just imagine. This is what working with a coach can bring you.

This professional is a personal coach. You may hire a counsellor, therapist, mentor or private tutor who provides some aspects of the above. Alternatively, you may have a colleague who informally coaches you, or a preceptor or mentor through a formalised mentoring structure. Someone who helps you grow by being there for you, listening, questioning and holding you accountable is a coach.

How people use their coaches

Some people hire a coach for a while, to 'jump start' them, point them in the right direction, and then continue alone. Some people hire coaches during challenging periods. Others work regularly with a coach. This may be the same coach over a number of years or they may switch coaches to get a flavour of different coaching styles and have different input.

Much of what we understand about this 'maturation' process, or the process of personal growth, comes from the field of psychotherapy and the professional who has traditionally been called upon to offer support in this area has been the psychotherapist. Unfortunately, due to the stigma which so often accompanies 'therapy', people often don't feel comfortable to consult a therapist unless there is a serious problem: unless things are going seriously wrong. Effective coaching has the potential to be, in effect, a 'psychological' inoculation. Coaching offers a way for each of us to access valuable support for ourselves during the process of growth, and to equip ourselves with valuable life skills before our lives start going wrong. It is closer to prevention than cure, as it can equip us with the psychological tools to avoid 'problems'.

The rise of the personal coach

We live in changing times. Our generation has had to deal with the rate of such change. We are experiencing change in our homes, our workplaces, and our relationships at an unprecedented rate. We consume things quicker, change our furniture faster, our cars, televisions, entertainment equipment, our technology increases faster, we are constantly learning how to operate our new microwave, video, CD player, DVD player, mobile phone, cordless phone or computer. We switch jobs frequently and often learn a new skill set with each role. The pace of life and desire to find the best jobs means we move home with more frequency. We are learning at an exponential rate which means we are not steadily progressing along a consistent learning curve – the curve is getting progressively steeper.

We even change our relationships more frequently. We are more likely to divorce and re-marry than previous generations and we divorce and re-marry at a faster rate. We are likely to have had a series of relationships in our lifetimes. With this we also need to learn new skills in relating to others and handling our emotions. We need an advanced emotional, interpersonal, 'relating' skill set. Emotional intelligence (EQ) is an umbrella term used to describe emotional maturity and advanced interpersonal, relating and communicating skills.

Concurrent with rapid change and technological advancement has been an increasing social isolation. Over the last 50 years, people have participated in fewer and fewer group activities and opt more for home entertainments and leisure pursuits which rarely, if ever, stretch them outside of their familiar friends and family. When I was in post as a Community Midwife, I observed how isolated many new mothers on large modern housing estates seemed to be. On any weekday these large residential estates became 'ghost towns', with most people out at work and school. I visited many women with newborn infants who lived over one hour's drive away from their nearest relatives and whose partner, friends and neighbours were out at work all day.

The ease with which information is readily available, coupled with the fact that people have more disposable income, has meant that for this generation personal growth and lifelong learning is an affordable choice. The training and education industries are also undergoing rapid change making ongoing learning more accessible than ever. There are now more options than ever before for continued learning, ranging from teleclasses (classes held over the telephone using teleconferencing facilities) to greater options for education including distance learning. People are appreciating that learning is valuable, that they can do it themselves, at home, and that it need not be expensive. More than ever before, people are open to the idea that they don't have to settle for what they have, and that it is acceptable to try and reach for something better.

Life coaches are coaching people in the personal, professional and social skills they need to stay ahead in this fast-paced ever-changing society. These include career management skills, financial management skills, business management skills, personal management skills (health, wellbeing, personal effectiveness) and relationship skills.

Do you need a coach?

When I first began my coaching practice many people said to me: 'I don't need a coach, I don't have any problems.' Soon, I would hear this same person saying: 'I need a holiday!'

Only a few years ago, during the middle of the 20th century, a holiday was considered something of a luxury, available only to a few people who could afford it. Now it is seen as a 'need', which must be met as part of our strategy for maintaining optimum health. At the time of writing, personal or life coaching is either viewed as a luxury for the few who can afford it, for companies to reward their top executives, or as a substitute to 'therapy' for 'weak and needy' people who cannot figure things out for themselves. This rather limiting viewpoint is changing fast as more people have personal experience of coaching and appreciate the value coaching can bring directly to them.

Whether you see any value in hiring a personal coach for yourself depends largely on how highly you value your own personal growth and development. If you are the sort of person who values personal growth, and is willing to choose and fund an educational course for yourself, you would probably appreciate and value working with a coach. However, if you only attend seminars when your employer sponsors you to go on work-related courses, and you see no intrinsic value to you personally, then you would probably not see any value in hiring a personal coach either. Do you choose to work on your growth for YOU, or do you see it only as a boring but necessary aspect of your career development?

COACHING MODELS

There are basically two coaching models from which all the others arise. The traditional view of coaching, in terms of instructing someone in a specific skill set, is known as directive coaching, in which specific guidance and instruction is given to the coachee. This is the model that is similar to tuition. The model of coaching which is widely advocated in business, and from which personal and life coaching stems, is the non-directive model. This is the contemporary model, where the coach does not give specific instruction but rather initiates the process of inquiry that leads to the coachee creating her own solutions.

Management coach model

Coaching aims to enhance the performance and learning ability of others. It involves providing feedback, but it also uses other techniques such as motivation, effective questioning and consciously matching your management style to the coachee's readiness to undertake a particular task.

(Landsberg,1996)

Management coaching is probably where coaching first ventured off the sports field and into the corporate world. Managers began to see benefits from coaching their staff rather than dictating or even instructing them. Influenced by inspirational, transformational and motivational psychology, and the increased use of organisational psychology in businesses and organisations, what was originally seen as a skill set or management tool is now increasingly being adopted as a management style. (For more on coaching as a management style see Chapter 6.)

Performance-centred coach model

Coaching in many contexts is related directly to performance. This is especially the case where employers hire either internal or external coaches to help staff achieve measurable results, such as increased sales, within an organisation or department.

Personal coaching

Since coaching is becoming established as a profession in its own right, many coaches have private clients, in addition to their corporate clients, in their coaching practices. Indeed, many coaches now choose to work with private clients alone, and do not do any corporate work. For many reasons, people are choosing to hire themselves a personal coach to overcome personal challenges, give themselves an edge in the career stakes, have greater clarity and/or focus and have more balance in their lives between life and work.

Life coaching

Life coaching is a form of personal coaching. Some coaches simply choose the term Life Coach (as I do) because it reflects the approach of coaching the whole person and focuses on upgrading their quality of life in all areas: physical, mental, spiritual and emotional.

Holistic coaching

As above, holistic (whole person) coaching takes a whole system view which focuses on the whole person. It is based on the philosophy that we are whole, all of the areas of our lives are interconnected, so making a change in one area will have repercussions for the whole system, body or person. This is interesting to consider both at a personal and organisational level. What affects one part of us affects all of us. For example, if your finances are a mess, what are the implications for all the other areas of your life? Is it possible to isolate one area of your life and not have it affect all the other areas? (See Chapter 7 for reference to taking a whole-system view of the NHS as an organisation.)

Co-active coaching

The term 'co-active' refers to the co-creative, partnership, nature of the coaching relationship. Effective non-directive coaching is co-active in that both coach and coachee are active participants in the co-creation of results and solutions for the coachee.

The term co-active refers to the fundamental nature of a coaching relationship in which the coach and client are active collaborators. In co-active coaching, this relationship is an alliance between two equals for the purpose of meeting the client's needs.

(Whitworth, Kimsey-House and Sandahl, 1998)

EXERCISE

Creating a model of coaching for healthcare

What would be an appropriate and effective model of coaching for healthcare?

What, in your experience, works?

Directive or non-directive?

Performance-centred?

How would such a relationship be structured?

What elements would be essential?

What would you include, and what would you leave out?

How would a coach be allocated or chosen?

Would you be able to choose a coach from among your peers and role models?

Would you be allocated an allowance, or learning grant, to hire your own external coach?

Take a blank piece of paper and spend 20 minutes listing the qualities that you would find beneficial in a coaching relationship.

(I am keen to hear your experience of this exercise. If you are willing, please e-mail your feedback to ruth@dreamcoach.co.uk)

COACHING STYLES AND FOCUS

Process coaching

Process coaching is a style of coaching where the coach focuses mainly on listening, supporting, empathising and 'being with' a coachee who is going through a challenging time. This is a challenging coaching style, and not all coaches are happy to offer this. Being comfortable with silence is essential while coachees think through their issues or experience their feelings. The focus is one of support and being with a coachee who is sorting out and observing their thoughts, feelings and emotions. This way, the coachee is able to view her situation from within and experience it. This is experiential learning. The coachee may arrive at a state of acceptance, or may not. She may create her own solutions, or not. It is the coachee's agenda. It is her experience. It is her learning process.

Process coaching allows clients to fully be in their experience rather than talk about their experience on a superficial level, or try to talk their way around it or talk themselves out of it.

(Whitworth, Kimsey-House and Sandahl, 1998)

Fulfilment coaching

Many people hire a personal coach because they want a sense of direction or meaning in their lives. In fulfilment coaching, the focus of the coaching is on first identifying the coachee's core values and beliefs before identifying what action they need to take to align their lives with their values, give their lives more meaning and feel fulfilled.

Balance coaching

One of the biggest challenges for many of us today is how to strike a balance between work and home commitments. Often we feel permanently guilty. When we are at home we feel guilty because there is something we should be doing at work, and when we are at work we feel guilty because there is inevitably something more we should be doing at home. Some coaches specialise in coaching in this field of work-life balance. The busier we are, the more important it is that we develop excellent self-management skills.

Strategy coaching

As the name suggests, the coaching focus is on developing a strategy of how to get from A to B. Again, this is most often associated with corporate coaching but it is evident also in personal coaching where coachees have a sense of where they want to go but not how to get there. Hiring a coach brings a partner into the situation to brainstorm the advantages and disadvantages, throw new ideas into the pot, and co-create a strategy. This can be used for any long-term planning: career, financial, business are but a few examples.

Situational coaching

This is where the coaching focuses on the coachee's situation. An example is 'stress management' coaching, which focuses just on one area of the coachee's life, namely managing their stress.

> *Stress Management Coaching (SMC) is the name we are using for a one-to-one 'talking' intervention aimed at helping a non-clinical population take an active, problem-solving approach to dealing with the causes of the various behavioural, psychological and physiological difficulties popularly associated with the term 'stress'. SMC is psycho-educational in approach, includes the teaching of coping strategies, and is similar to one-to-one training.*
>
> *(Smith and Palmer, 2000)*

Specialist coaching

In addition to the holistic coaches mentioned above, there are many specialisms within personal coaching. There are coaches who specialise in coaching areas such as empowerment, self-esteem and confidence building. Some coaches specialise in coaching people in financial management or new business start-ups. Others specialise in coaching public speaking, health and fitness and/or weight loss.

Coaching is a powerful process in which the synergy of the coach-coachee relationship benefits the coachee by motivating, empowering and facilitating personal growth. Coaching in one form or another has always been with us, and in a sense is nothing new. The 'new' trend is that coaching is currently evolving into a distinct and separate discipline in addition to being a skill set which can be applied by anyone. There is benefit in both of these areas for healthcare practitioners and our clients. We can both develop a coaching skill set, which will enable us to coach our clients, and hire our own personal coach to facilitate personal and professional development.

Where coaching is used effectively, it benefits our working environment by helping us look at how we relate to one another, how effective we are, how we develop our leadership skills and how we interact with our colleagues and clients. Coaching has huge potential in changing the culture of an organisation which is essential for the continued growth and survival of our health service. Whittemore et al (2002) applied coaching in a healthcare context to facilitate lifestyle change in diabetic patients. Her nurse-coaching intervention consisted of facilitation, education, psychosocial support and motivational guidance.

A coach for all seasons?

Is there such a thing as a universal coach? A coach who can work with you and grow with you? Or will you find that one coach coaches you on one aspect of your development, while another coach is better on another area? Individual coaches are unique, each with different styles. If you find the 'right' coach for you, meaning that you work well together and you make progress with this coach, you may choose to stay with this coach for as long as you are making progress.

If coaching is not working for you, it is important that you try another coach with a completely different style. Since the synergy of the relationship is important for coaching to be effective, you may need to literally 'shop around' to find the coach that is perfect for you.

DISTINCTIONS

Already we can see areas of overlap between coaching and teaching, coaching and therapy, coaching and mentoring and even coaching and midwifery or nursing. In practice it may not be clear to us when we are coaching and when we are mentoring. There are skills which transfer easily from one role to another, such as listening skills. As with many new disciplines it helps to create a distinction between the roles.

Coaching and mentoring

How does coaching differ from mentoring? Mentoring is task focused. The focus in mentoring is on what you do and how well you do it. In mentoring, your performance is the focus. In coaching, your performance may improve as a result of your being coached, but not because the coach focused on what it is you are doing. Your mentor focuses on what you are doing, why you are doing it, how you are doing it and how you can do it better. In coaching, the coach focuses on you and where your attention is, what you are feeling, what your experience is and what you notice about you. Mentoring focuses on what you do, coaching focuses on who you are.

Coaching and teaching

In a sense, a coach is simply a facilitator of learning. The coach creates a nurturing environment in which the coachee discovers the very best within herself. Where teaching is facilitative and non-directional rather than instructional it is very akin to coaching. I have no doubt that the best teachers are also coaches and draw upon coaching skills in their work. Gallwey (1997) is often attributed with introducing the non-directive element into coaching. It is also suggested (Whitmore, 1996) that his influence has transformed sports coaching from instruction to non-directive coaching. It comes as no surprise then that Gallwey's background was in education and, more specifically, person-centred, non-directive, facilitative education. He shifted the emphasis from the teaching of sport to developing the potential of the player. Gallwey recognised that people, especially adults, learn best by observing how well they are doing and discovering the answers for themselves rather than being told.

Most learning is not the result of instruction. It is rather the result of unhampered participation in a meaningful setting.

(Illich, 1971, p.44)

The coach sets up the environment in which learning takes place and helps the coachee to identify and remove obstacles, and interference, so the coachee's natural growth and learning may proceed unimpeded.

Coaching is the art of helping others to reach their potential. A coach may be inspiring, guiding, motivating, informing, instructing, teaching, mentoring, advising, listening, directing, non-directing, strategising, co-creating, educating and/or empowering. It depends on the coach's background and skill set and what the coachee requires of a coaching relationship. Coaching works by direct interaction with the coachee. Enhancing coachees' confidence and belief in their own ability, and expanding their potential. As the coachee reaches and exceeds her own limitations she sets new goals for herself and sets about reaching those. The coachee's 'potential' is infinite as her ability becomes dynamic: growing, expanding and constantly changing.

Coaching differs from teaching significantly, in that the coach need not have any knowledge of the coachee's chosen subject other than a knowledge of how to coach.

Coaching and therapy

Among similar professions, coaching is probably most often compared with therapy. It is not always easy to see clearly defined lines between what constitutes suitable material for coaching and what should be referred to a therapist. Unless she possesses appropriate qualifications, a coach is not usually qualified or competent to make medical or mental health diagnoses. It is not the coach's role. However, coaches do focus on their coachees' feelings and emotions, so how do we distinguish between coaching and psychotherapy?

Coaching focuses on building strengths, on discovering and nurturing talent, then adding the skills and knowledge required to capitalise on it (see Chapter 3). Therapy, by definition, focuses on 'what's wrong' and 'fixing'. They are very different standpoints.

The difference is one of sickness and health. As part of the overall process, a coach may sometimes (though not always) focus on emotional growth and maturity in healthy individuals. This is always as an adjunct to, rather than as the sole focus of, coaching and coaches never diagnose or apply treatments with the intention to effect a 'cure'. As we saw in the earlier definition of stress management coaching, coaching is:

a one-to-one 'talking' intervention aimed at helping a non-clinical population take an active, problem-solving approach to dealing with the causes of the various behavioural, psychological and physiological difficulties.

(Smith and Palmer, 2000)

Coaching offers a way for us to nurture healthy emotional development without having to frame ourselves within a sickness model. It gives us permission, within a structured professional format, to look at how we can develop our emotions. A gardener gives as much attention to his healthy plants as he does to his sick ones.

It is also important to differentiate between emotional order and disorder. Therapists work with mental illness and emotional disorder; coaches work with normal, healthy, emotional growth (amongst other things).

Often there can be a coaching approach to what was previously considered a therapy issue. Consider the example of stress management. Stress is a part of normal life in this busy world. If we need help in developing extra skills in order to help us learn to manage our stress, does this necessarily make us ill?

Yet we may have experienced stress to a degree that we suffer from stress-related illness, such as Post Traumatic Stress Disorder. It may be the case that we have become ill as a result of stress, and that we need therapy until we become well again. At which point coaching can certainly help us learn to manage our stress to prevent us becoming ill again. During 'dips' into illness, coaching may continue in conjunction with therapy, if the client is well enough to participate.

It has been the tradition to classify anything remotely linked to our emotional competencies, or lack thereof, as 'illness' requiring therapeutic solutions. According to Peck:

> *Few of us can escape being neurotic or character disordered to at least some degree (which is why essentially everyone can benefit from psychotherapy if he or she is seriously willing to participate in the process).*
>
> *(Peck, 1990)*

Yet, even among therapists, there is an acknowledgement that what they are witnessing is part of normal, healthy, emotional growth and maturity (Lerner, 1989; Rogers, 1961). The current trend is towards acknowledging that our emotional domain is simply another aspect of development, in which we can learn core skills at any age. Emotional intelligence (EQ) is currently being taught in some pioneering schools, either as an adjunct to, or inherent within, the usual curriculum (Goleman, 1996).

Routinely framing our emotional development within the context of illness leads us to view any emotional issues as problematic and to frame them in a 'sickness' context. Anything relating to our emotions becomes viewed as 'abnormal', a weakness or unhealthy.

Does this mean that we are experiencing an epidemic of mental illness? Or that mental illness is endemic in our society? Or is it rather that the concept of illness does not fit our pattern of emotional growth? Perhaps it is inadequate as a context within which to describe our emotional experience and growth. If we are not ill, why would we seek therapeutic solutions? We may be witnessing a stage in our evolution as a society that can be facilitated like any other stage of growth. As a species, we are continually evolving and our emotional development is part of that. We are learning how to relate to one another, and to our emotions, in a completely new way.

Coaches are filling a gap in the health market. Healthy intelligent people, who know they want to grow emotionally and handle all their relationships more maturely both at home and at work, are seeking out personal coaches to help them. They do not want to be told they are deficient or ill. They do not want to be psychoanalysed. They are seeking someone who will partner them in a journey of self-exploration leading to personal growth.

As we move as a society from a sickness/cure model towards a health/prevention model we look towards a profession which facilitates growth and change rather than a therapeutic model to 'cure' our 'illness'. Teaching springs to mind, yet we are not requiring specific information. We look for someone to facilitate, encourage, inspire and motivate us as we co-create our new way of being. As we undertake a paradigm shift from sickness to health, as we create a new way of relating to one another, as we learn the steps to a new interpersonal dance, the word 'coach' fits perfectly to describe this new professional role.

2

The psychology of coaching

There is nothing either good or bad but thinking makes it so.

William Shakespeare

This chapter outlines some of the psychological theories that lend themselves to explaining how the coaching process works. This will hopefully give us an understanding of why coaching is often effective and why, sometimes, it is not.

The psychology of coaching is the psychology of human growth. How we, as human beings, grow, learn, develop and realise our potential. What factors enhance, nurture and accelerate our growth? What factors impede and inhibit our growth? What motivates us?

The coaching process is not fully understood. There are huge gaps in our theoretical knowledge. Until recently, our knowledge base of human psychology was informed by the therapeutic professions. Psychoanalysts looked at 'what was wrong' and 'how to fix it' rather than focusing on what works.

A HIERARCHY OF NEED

Some psychologists have studied the psychology of 'success': they studied healthy individuals and put their attention on behaviour that was already working successfully. Maslow (1982) suggested we are motivated by an inner drive to meet our needs, and that

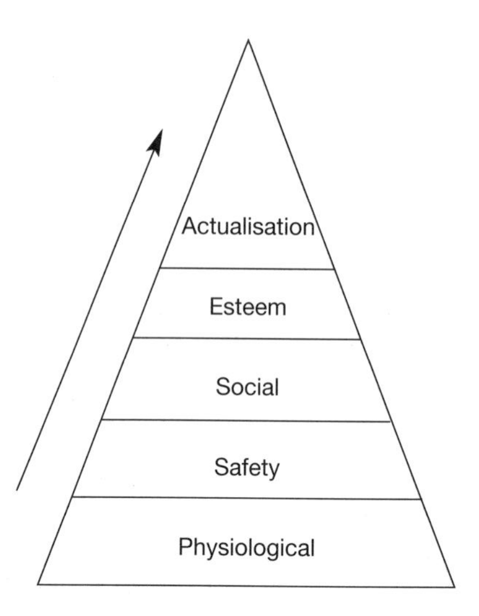

Figure 2.1 Maslow's hierarchy of human needs

our needs are hierarchical in nature. According to Maslow we progress from meeting our physiological needs toward self-actualisation (see Figure 2.1). We will always be motivated to meet the need that has the highest priority. So, for example, we will not consider our safety until we have met our physiological needs, and we will not consider our social needs until we have met our need for safety.

Coaches are interested in needs because needs can be obstacles to our growth. Maslow noticed that if we are both hungry and thirsty, our attention will be focused on our need to drink and we will not even think about food until our thirst is quenched. This is because we will die of thirst before we will die of hunger. This illustrates how we are driven by our most immediate need. From a coaching point of view, needs are important because they are a major distraction to the coachee and a drain on energy. Nothing else can have our coachee's full attention until their needs are met. As Maslow suggested, we cannot consider our social needs until we feel safe. If, for example, we have a coachee who desires to develop a supportive social network, yet they have a fear of losing their job and their home, we can see how they will be driven by their need for safety before they will be able to turn their full attention to their social needs. As a coach, we guide the client in meeting their most immediate need so that they are free to turn their attention to what they desire.

PERSONAL NEEDS AND VALUES

If we have unmet needs, they will drive us until they are met. An example with which we are all familiar is that of needing to go to the toilet. No matter what you are doing, if you have an overriding need to go and empty your bladder it will dominate your thoughts and actions until you've taken care of it. It's much the same with personal needs. If you have unmet personal needs they will drive you until they are met and will take your energy and attention off everything else.

Basic needs such as food, water, warmth, shelter and love are common to us all. The higher up Maslow's hierarchy we get, the more our needs become personal and individual. So what is a need for one is not necessarily a need for someone else. This leads to judgement – often of ourselves. We may feel 'bad' about ourselves for needing something, yet personal needs are just as important as basic needs. We are naturally drawn towards self-actualisation and we cannot attain this while we have unmet needs. If we have a need for touch, closeness, to be held, we will not be our best until this need is met. We will not be the best version of who we can be.

One day during the early 1980s I was walking along Otterspool Promenade in Liverpool with a friend from Cologne, Germany. The promenade runs along the bank of the River Mersey. My friend commented on the degree of pollution and filth in the river at that time. (This was prior to the Mersey basin clean-up initiatives; I am pleased to say that the River Mersey is now vastly improved and is a haven to wildlife.) She was shocked and asked how we could allow this damage to our river. It was a thought-provoking question. How could we? The answer lies in Maslow's theory of needs, and the relative poverty of Liverpool at that time. Liverpool featured highly on the Department of the Environment deprivation index (Department of the Environment, 1995) as one of the most economically deprived areas in Western Europe. When people are worried about where their next meal is coming from, or how to keep a roof over their heads, they have little time to worry about what is happening with the river. This illustrates how unmet needs can block growth and development on a social scale.

Within the coaching relationship it is the coachee rather than the coach who is responsible for identifying their needs. The coach's role is to use the coaching process of inquiry and skilled questioning to enable the coachee to realise where her needs are, and to distinguish between needs and values. This is often easier said than done and, again, it is the coachee who will ultimately make this distinction.

The distinction between needs and values is not clear by any means. What may be a need for one person can be a value for another and vice-versa. As a rule, needs drive us while values attract us. Needs push and values pull. It is the difference between the proverbial carrot and stick. Our values pull us towards them. We are inexplicably drawn towards them and we feel fulfilled when we can live and work in accord with them. Needs drive us. We are driven until they are met. We do not necessarily gain satisfaction, fulfillment or pleasure from them. Indeed, sometimes we feel anxious and under 'pressure', yet we are driven to acquire whatever it is we need. This is easy to understand when we think of basic needs such as food, water, sleep and a home. When we are driven to meet our higher needs it becomes harder to understand that they are still simply something that we need in order to be the best of who we are.

Needs become personal the higher up Maslow's hierarchy we progress (Figure 2.1). Physiological needs are common to us all. We easily identify with the need for food, water, warmth and shelter, but when it comes to what we may need in order to have a sense of self-esteem and self-actualisation, this will vary between individuals. Because of this, there is a tendency for us to feel guilt. We sometimes feel it is wrong to need something that others do not, and we may sometimes lack understanding of others who need things we do not.

We sometimes meet people who seem very 'needy'. We do not feel comfortable being around needy people. We notice how needy people drain our energy, and when it is us who are needy, we feel drained all the time. Yet we are unable to define what it is that makes us uncomfortable around such people. What is 'neediness'? We experience a vague idea that these people need something from us in some way. Often what we are detecting is an unconscious personal need for acceptance, approval, love or acknowledgement. If we are able to identify our personal needs, so that we become consciously aware of them, we can take steps to meet them so that we do not appear 'needy' to others.

The distinction between needs and values is personal. My example was living in the countryside. While I loved living in the city, with access to the restaurants, entertainment, theatres and bars – all the facilities a city has to offer – I always longed for the country. I felt just as at home in a field, walking my dogs, as I did in a restaurant. I believed it to be a value, in that I knew I loved the country and intended to retire there. I walked in the country at weekends and eventually bought a caravan in the countryside. It was not enough. I became increasingly depressed upon my return to the city and increasingly despaired at the 'concrete jungle'. We finally made a decision not to wait until retirement but to move as soon as we could. That was in 1998. It was only after we moved that I realised how much my desire to live in the country was a personal need for me. I need solitude, the relaxed, unhurried, environment and to be close to nature, in order to be my best. Needing to 'live in the country' may not seem like a need to you, yet it illustrates precisely what, in coaching, we mean by a need. In coaching we define a need as any condition which must be met in order for you to be at your best.

EXERCISE

Part 1:
Take 10 minutes to reflect on what you feel you really need in order to be your very best. Write for 20-30 minutes without stopping. Don't edit what you write or tell yourself 'it's silly' or 'not allowed' for some reason. Just write what you feel you really need. Make a list.

Part 2:
Choose five needs from your list and ask yourself:

What would need to happen to ensure these needs are met permanently?

(I am keen to hear your experience of this exercise. If you are willing, please e-mail your feedback to ruth@dreamcoach.co.uk)

A PSYCHOLOGY OF SELF

Rogers (1961) observed a trend towards self-definition in most of his patients. He suggests that, provided we are healthy, and are in a conducive, nurturing environment, we naturally tend towards growth and learning. It is what humans want to do. When we do not, it is because some other factor is stifling our growth. Remove the obstacles to growth, provide the right environment and people will explore and learn all of their own accord. He suggested we are in a process of developing a clear sense of self and becoming more fully who we really are. Rogers calls this a maturation process.

Some coaches (myself included) request that coachees keep a coaching journal, or diary, in which to record their own observations of themselves. This assists in developing our sense of self, our sense of who we are as unique individuals.

Rogers also emphasised the importance of unconditional positive regard as being essential to the creation of a nurturing environment for growth and learning. This is also sometimes referred to as a 'non-judgemental' approach. It is difficult not to make judgements, we all do, yet unconditional positive regard calls for us to hold our clients in high regard whether we are of the same opinion as them or not. This is the essence of humanistic psychology: the principle that we can hold every other human being in high positive regard merely by virtue of the fact that they are another human being. The unconditional element challenges us to hold people in high regard even when they demonstrate actions or behaviours with which we cannot agree and do not condone. This means there are no conditions attached to our regard for them. In coaching, this is essential. The implied message is:

I hold you in high esteem regardless of whether you do your fieldwork or not, whether you reach your goals or not, and whether you continue coaching or not. You cannot say, do, or fail to do anything that will affect my positive regard for you as a person.

This does not mean that you agree with or condone their actions: as we will see later (Chapter 3), coaching is even more powerful when the coach has an opinion and can express it directly and with compassion.

POSITIVE EXPECTATIONS

When the coach has positive expectations of the client, the client rises to meet them. This phenomenon is not fully understood and is often referred to as the 'halo' effect. The halo effect is where our positive impression of someone becomes fulfilled in reality.

Coaches hold their coachees in high esteem and positive regard; in addition, they consciously have higher expectations of them than they would of themselves. By receiving encouragement to always beat their own record and surpass their previous 'best', the coachee grows and realises her potential.

The coach often uses language such as 'what I want for you is...' to express an expectation they have for the coachee. This is not a random statement but is normally related to an implied or explicit ambition that the coachee has for themselves. The coach will take the coachee's vision and add to it, exceeding their expectations of themselves.

SYNERGY

Coaching works because of the synergy between coach and coachee. Synergy is the combined effect that is greater than the sum of the two individual effects. This means that something greater occurs than would occur if the two individuals worked separately from each other and then combined their results. The coach and coachee form a team or partnership. Coachees use the coach as a 'sounding board' to test ideas, and the coach brings his or her own ideas, experience and wisdom to the table. Many more choices are generated than there would be by either individual alone (see Figure 2.2).

Life coaching is client-centred, which means the client (the coachee) always sets the agenda. The coaching session focuses only on the coachee's vision, mission, purpose, goals, strategy, planning action and on overcoming barriers, obstacles and challenges which might be in the way.

REMOVING OBSTACLES

In order to achieve any goal in life, we need to have some way to deal with whatever is in our way. Often it is ourselves. Fear is a big issue for many of us. For example, sometimes we do not even apply for a job or promotion that we would love because we either fear we would not succeed (fear of failure), or we fear going through the process of application and interview (fear of discomfort, resistance). Part of the coach's role is to help us identify what holds us back and to help us overcome our fears.

How does coaching work?

Coaching creates a safe space where you can think, reflect, plan, play, experiment, learn, discover, create and take bolder action than you ever thought you could. This happens through:

Teamwork: My clients and I become a team. I become your partner. You can use me as a 'sounding board' to test your ideas. I will sometimes bring my ideas to the table to give you more choices.

Focus: You, as my client, always set the agenda. We focus only on your goals and on creating the strategy for you to achieve them.

Structure: You refine, define and set your goals. We identify what is needed to bridge the gap between where you are now and where you want to be. We break the 'big' goals down into 'do-able' pieces. We do this within a timescale. Within this structure your dreams can become reality.

Commitment: You make a personal commitment to achieving your goals. Then you commit yourself to whatever steps are necessary to make them a reality.

Accountability: There is something about sharing your plans with another person that makes you more likely to stick to them. It somehow strengthens your resolve.

Self-management: You manage yourself well. This means developing and maintaining systems to ensure your personal effectiveness, health, well-being, personal finances, home, car, relationships with others and much more! There's probably a lot more to managing YOU than you realise!

Momentum: Checking in with your coach at regular periods by telephone and e-mail helps you to stay focused on your goals and keeps the energy and momentum going.

Action-learning: The weekly coaching call is only the beginning. The real learning takes place in between calls as you take action, make changes in your life, then reflect and learn from those actions which are more or less successful – for you.

Adapted frm internet document located at: http://www.dreamcoach.co.uk/FAQ.html

Figure 2.2 How does coaching work?

SELF-ESTEEM

Making a commitment to ourselves, and being prepared to keep it, involves valuing ourselves enough to feel we deserve it. Low self-esteem can be an obstacle which prevents us having the persistence required to pursue our dreams. Sometimes our negative core beliefs are reflected in language statements such as: 'There is no point in trying, I never win.'

We may never say such statements out loud, yet they can be part of an ongoing negative internal dialogue. If left unchallenged, this becomes a self-fulfilling prophecy. Part of the coaching process involves empowering coachees to a greater degree of self-efficacy; that is, the belief that they are in control of events and can control their own future.

COGNITIVE BEHAVIOURAL APPROACH

Coaching is distinct from cognitive behavioural therapy (see Chapter 1: coaching and therapy) yet some coaching styles, such as process coaching, adopt a cognitive behavioural approach to challenge a coachee's fixed behaviour patterns. This approach is especially effective in improving self-esteem and confidence.

A central theme in coaching is that we can do what we believe we can, and cannot do what we believe we cannot. What we believe makes a crucial difference to the outcome. Coaches will encourage us to examine any beliefs we hold about ourselves which may be limiting us and preventing us from achieving our desired outcomes.

Most of us are aware at some time or another that we have negative thoughts, yet we may be completely unaware that our thoughts have any connection to how we feel and what we believe about our own ability. In this approach the coach encourages the coachee to become aware of thoughts which are negative and self-critical and to challenge our thoughts. Often our thoughts reflect underlying assumptions we have made, perhaps years earlier, which have been left unchallenged.

Brendgen (2002) explains that the cognitive behavioural approach is based on three premises:

- we feel the way we think
- most bad feelings come from illogical thoughts or distortions, and
- we can change the way we feel.

Since it is the coach's role to enable the coachee to mature and grow, it is also part of the coach's role to encourage the coachee to challenge negative and limiting thoughts. The coach encourages the coachee to put her thoughts to the test, to subject her own thoughts to inquiry. As an example, we may notice considerable negative self-talk and self-criticism in the coachee's language. We would draw this to her attention and maybe set some fieldwork or make a request (see coaching skills, Chapter 3) that they notice this and write down their self-observations in their coaching journal. In this instance, we would be encouraging the coachee to first notice her thoughts, to develop a degree of self-awareness. Challenging the validity of her thoughts would come later and such challenging would be done by the coachee herself, with the help of her coach.

Goleman (1996) describes 'depressogenic' thought which, if allowed to go unchallenged, is responsible for depression. He points to a growing body of evidence that suggests that even moderate to severe clinical depression can be reversed and prevented by developing a self-awareness of thought patterns and coaching people in techniques which challenge their thinking.

Katie (2002) developed a simple process of inquiry to challenge our thoughts, based on her observation that it is not the thought itself, but rather our attachment to our thoughts, that creates our discomfort. She has created a simple, yet effective, inquiry process which can be used by anyone using the same four questions:

1. *Is it true?*
2. *Can you absolutely know that it is true?*
3. *How do you react when you think that thought?*
4. *Who would you be without the thought?*

(Katie, 2002)

(Worksheets and full instructions on using this inquiry process are available from Byron Katie's website at: http://www.thework.com)

This approach is extremely effective where the aim of coaching is to build the coachee's self-esteem and confidence. Core negative beliefs can be effectively challenged so that the coachee re-orientates around a new concept of reality. We may hold negative core beliefs such as:

I'm no good.

I'm a failure.

No one will ever love me.

I am a waste of space.

Through identification of the lie behind the thoughts and developing a strong, action-oriented methodology for change, the third premise of the model is addressed, i.e. you can change the way you feel.

(Brendgen, 2002)

EXERCISE

Write down some of your own negative core beliefs.

Notice who you become when you think like that. Notice how you react. How do you feel? How does it make you behave when you believe that? For example, do you shrink inside? Do your shoulders slump?

(I am keen to hear your experience of this exercise. If you are willing, please e-mail your feedback to ruth@dreamcoach.co.uk)

COGNITIVE DISSONANCE

We can see that, if we believe we will never come to any good, this becomes a self-fulfilling prophesy. This happens because we actually act out our 'bad' behaviour to support the view that we ARE bad. This is not a conscious choice, but rather the effect of what Festinger (1957) terms cognitive dissonance. He suggested that people experience dissonance when two of their cognitions (thoughts, feelings, beliefs) are contradictory, and that this dissonance is extremely uncomfortable. Festinger and Carlsmith (1959) demonstrated that, since a state of dissonance is too uncomfortable to bear, people would even change their fundamental beliefs and attitudes to reduce cognitive dissonance. This drive to reduce cognitive dissonance at any cost explains otherwise seemingly irrational behaviour. Why would any of us choose to be bad? Yet we will do anything to reconcile our belief with our actions, and reduce cognitive dissonance, so if we believe we are bad we must act bad.

Byron Katie (2002) occasionally works with hardened criminals in prison, some of whom are under sentence of death or life imprisonment. She uses her inquiry process to affirm and acknowledge them, challenging their long-held belief that they are intrinsically 'bad':

I love thanking these men for sacrificing their entire lives to teach our children how not to live – and therefore how to live – if they want to be free. I tell them that they are the greatest teachers and that their lives are good and needed. Before I leave, I ask them, 'Would you spend the rest of your life in prison if you knew it would keep one child from having to live what you're living?' And many of these violent men understand, and they just well up with tears...

(Katie, 2002)

NEURO LINGUISTIC PROGRAMMING

Neuro Linguistic Programming (NLP) is a term used to describe a group of specific psychological approaches to changing thought patterns and language, with the aim of improving performance, personal effectiveness and controlling emotions. Similarly to the methods already mentioned, NLP draws our attention to the way our thoughts and language influence our beliefs and actions. With its origins in hypnosis, NLP focuses on changing thought and language to change our belief and action. Some coaches specialise in using NLP techniques.

STRUCTURE AND STRATEGY

The coachee refines, defines and sets her goals. Coachee and coach form a partnership together to identify what is needed to bridge the gap between where the coachee is now and where she wants to be. Then they co-create a strategy. The strategy is not fixed in stone, it evolves; however, it is an important starting point. To achieve anything, we need a framework in which to work. Strategy gives us a framework within which we can begin to identify the stepping stones towards our goal. Such stepping stones can consist of some big goals, such as securing finances and purchasing or building premises. Coach and coachee then start to break the overwhelmingly 'big' goals down into manageable smaller goals. Taking a large goal such as 'securing finances', a brainstorming session between coach and coachee could generate many options and actions that can be taken towards this goal. The coachee would identify which feel appropriate for her, and then coach and coachee can come up with a daily action list. A daily action list is used to motivate the coachee towards a goal. Before creating the list, coach and client would identify which actions would, when taken consistently over time, lead to the goal being achieved. For example, if the goal was to call 100 sponsors and ask for their support, the identified daily action might be to call 10 sponsors every day for the next 10 days. In this example, the daily action list is the structure through which the goal will be met.

In setting goals, it is wise to consider the popular acronym which reminds us that goals should be SMART:

- Specific
- Measurable
- Achievable
- Relevant
- Time-oriented.

TIMEFRAMES AND COMMITMENT

It is important to design structure, actions and goals, within the context of a timescale. If the coachee commits to calling 10 people, her coach might say: 'Wonderful, when will you do it?'

This turns an idea into a firm commitment. Without this commitment to do x within a certain time or before a certain date, then it could just be left, forgotten about, 'put on the back burner', gradually fall lower and lower down the list of priorities until 'life' takes over and the coachee is right back where she started, wondering: 'That was a great idea, why didn't I ever do that?'

The time commitment ensures we keep whatever is important to us right at the top of our list of priorities, and provides the practical structure within which our pipedreams, visions, plans and ambitions will become reality. We can see that the structure is the practical framework, consisting of short-term goals, action steps and a timescale, within which we achieve our aims. This is also what provides clients with a sense of focus.

EXERCISE

Step 1:
Think of something important that you would like to achieve sometime in your life. Draw out your vision. What does it look like? What will it feel like when you are 'there'? What will it say about you? Be as specific and vivid as possible. Imagine yourself walking, talking, eating and sleeping in your vision. Touch, taste, feel, hear, see and smell it. Write or paint a representation of your vision and pin it up somewhere where you will see it every day.

Step 2:
Take a reality check. Look at your current reality. This might be uncomfortable, but take a good hard look anyway. Be honest with yourself. It is important to know where you are now. Identify the gap between where you are now and where you want to be.

Step 3:
Brainstorm. Call a friend and ask if they will 'play' this with you. Tell them your goal, and where you are now. Ask yourselves: 'What would need to happen to bridge this gap?'

Have fun exploring as many different options as possible. Keep it fast paced, fun and light. Don't dismiss anything at this stage. The ridiculous and impossible-sounding ideas are often more realistic than you would imagine. Record them all.

Step 4:
Look at the ideas generated in Step 3 (above) and see which feel right for you. Choose as many as you can feasibly pursue. Pick the one that appeals to you most, and agree to do it. Set a date by which you will have achieved it and mark it in your diary or calendar. When this is completed choose another, and repeat the process until you have completed all your goals.

(I am keen to hear your experience of this exercise. If you are willing, please e-mail your feedback to ruth@dreamcoach.co.uk)

STRENGTHS AND COMPETENCIES

Coaches empower people by focusing on their natural talent, strengths and competencies, rather than their weaknesses. Once a coach has identified a key strength, talent or competency in a coachee we acknowledge it. This means telling coachees that they have a strength, what it is that we have identified as a strength and acknowledging them for it. To receive acknowledgement from another is an empowering and validating experience.

Coaches have traditionally expressed concern in their coachees' self-belief since this has such an impact on our behaviour and performance. If Tim Henman does not absolutely believe that he can win Wimbledon, he will not. In addition to challenging limiting beliefs, self-doubt and instilling self-belief into the coachee, it is the coach's role to identify talent and nurture strengths. It is because of this aspect of the coaching role that many people mistakenly perceive coaching as simply 'cheerleading' or offering encouragement. Yet how do we distinguish between talent and a strength? Buckingham and Clifton (2002) define a strength as: 'consistent near perfect performance in an activity.' In contrast, talent is defined as: 'a special aptitude or faculty' (Pearsall and Trumble, 1996).

The philosophy of coaching is founded on truth and realism. Best practice in coaching would be to establish truth (or reality) by requesting the coachee take a measurement of some sort. Aptitude and consistency in performance are measurable qualities. Many coaches work with psychological profiles which give an indication toward a coachee's aptitude and strengths.

If someone hired a coach to help them become an opera singer, and they could not sing, a good coach would tell them so. This is different from having a coachee who believes they have no strengths in any area. This cannot be 'truth' or realism, any more than a coachee who believes they will excel at everything. Everyone has a strength. A simple test such as the Strengthsfinder Profile (Buckingham and Clifton, 2002) would reveal key areas and give some guidance to the kinds of activities in which this person could excel, given the skills and knowledge to add to their talent. Part of the initial coaching sessions might be a process of discovery, trying different things until the coachee finds what they like and have a natural flair for. Throughout the process, the coach may suggest many activities, some of which the coachee will shine at and some of which will not be appropriate. The coachee will always be learning something about themselves. During this process the coach may request that they keep a journal, and will certainly encourage them to pay attention to themselves. To what they felt good about, what they felt bad about, what helped them, what hindered them, etc.

In using psychological profiles, the coach is interested in discovering where we have a natural talent, tendency or flair, that can be built upon until it becomes a true strength. Coaching focuses on strengths in a society which often focuses on discovering our weaknesses and 'fixing' them. This is another contrast between coaching and therapy. By definition, therapy focuses on what is wrong with us that needs 'fixing' whereas coaching focuses on what is 'right' with us that can be developed.

THE FLOW STATE

In terms of performance, sports players often refer to being 'in the zone' They are talking about a 'flow state'. In terms of performance, a flow state is where we operate at the cutting edge of our own potential. When we are in a state of flow, we are working at the peak of our ability. We will be slightly challenged so that we are actually improving a little, yet we are still within the range of our ability to do so, our potential. If we are challenged too much we feel overwhelmed and our performance drops. If we are not challenged enough we become bored and, again, our performance falters. When we are in flow, we are improving, developing our ability, growing and stretching our potential. Meanwhile, to outside observers, we appear to make a complex task look quite easy. This is a sign of mastery in performance. When we witness someone making a task look easy, that we know is not, we are witnessing a flow state. A flow state in any field is necessary for fulfillment, growth and peak performance. This means striking the right balance between our feelings of overwhelm and boredom. Recognising what constitutes a 'flow state' for us requires a degree of self-awareness, a willingness to be honest with ourselves and courage to challenge ourselves. It is an important factor for our continued fulfilment and our sense of happiness or wellbeing.

EMOTIONAL INTELLIGENCE

As we develop greater awareness of our Self, we become more aware of our feelings. This is a crucial element in emotional intelligence or EQ (Emotional Quotient). Emotional intelligence incorporates a repertoire of interpersonal skills, self-awareness and control over our emotions. We may know of someone who is academically brilliant, yet totally inept when it comes to social skills.

Goleman (1996) suggests that, like IQ (cognitive Intelligence Quotient), EQ is quantifiable and we can measure specifically whether someone has high or low EQ. More importantly, it is suggested that EQ is not fixed. It can be improved, so that someone with low EQ can take action to raise their EQ.

EQ refers to a spectrum of life skills which includes social skills, communication and interpersonal skills and places equal emphasis on self-awareness and emotional control. How does this make a difference to our behaviour? Having self-awareness means not only knowing about ourselves, but being aware of how we feel in any given moment and knowing how to handle our emotions. Goleman (1996) suggests that until we possess a degree of self-awareness we remain prone to 'emotional hijacking' in which our emotions 'take over' and we have no control. It is the crucial difference between being swept along by a feeling rather than becoming aware of it. Until now it was largely assumed that some people possess greater 'self-control' than others by nature, and that 'self-control' is an inborn characteristic rather than a skill which can be learned. EQ brings the encouraging insight that rather than being helpless victims of our emotions we actually can develop control over them if we invest our time, attention and energy in learning how. The coaching process with its emphasis on self-awareness and action learning is an excellent tool for raising our EQ.

Coaching encourages the coachee to recognise 'choice points'. This means noticing the point at which we become aware that we are emotionally aroused, and where we have a choice. This sounds easier said than done and takes practice. The first step is to develop our self-awareness to the point where we recognise that we are emotionally aroused during the event rather than after the event. This means noticing how we tend to react or respond.

EXERCISE

As a piece of fieldwork I sometimes request that clients do this exercise comparing the words 'react' and 'respond' and contrasting the difference between the two. Take five minutes now and try this for yourself. Take a piece of A4-sized paper and draw a line down the middle, creating two columns. At the top of the first column write 'react' and at the top of the second column write 'respond'.

What do you notice about your answers?

(I am keen to hear your experience of this exercise. If you are willing, please e-mail your feedback to ruth@dreamcoach.co.uk)

Some of the distinctions that people make include: reacting is quick, automatic and knee-jerk whereas responding is slower, deliberate, more thought-out. I always point out that in doing this exercise we are not making it wrong to react, rather just noticing the difference, to gain clarity and be better informed about when it is appropriate to react and when it would be more appropriate to respond.

Goleman argues that a fast, knee-jerk reaction is always the result of a conditioned emotional response. The part of the brain which controls our emotional responses, the amygdala, has the ability to move us swiftly out of danger and, to ensure the response time is fast (it has been measured in nanoseconds, one billionth of a second), it by-passes our cognitive cortex in the process. Not only do we not think about it, we are unable to think about it, because the information has not been relayed to the cognitive (thinking, conscious) part of our brain, the cortex. If we put our hand on the iron and burn ourselves, we only become consciously aware of the fact after we have already removed ourselves from danger. We cannot imagine thinking in such a scenario. Consider how much physical damage would occur if we had to consciously think: 'I am aware my hand is burning – I will remove it from the heat now.'

Throughout our evolution, the amygdala has come to our rescue, ensuring we have an efficient 'fear: fight or flight' response to protect us from physical danger. It has the ability to weigh up a situation with lightening speed and, if it concludes that we are indeed in danger, the emotional response is triggered. The amygdala is extremely efficient in its stimulus-response reaction because it sacrifices accuracy for speed. It does not have time to relay information to the cortex then await the results of an analysis, so if a stimulus is similar enough to one that hurt you in the past, that is enough to warrant an emotional response from the amygdala. For a full description of the physiology, I recommend reading Goleman's description of the emotional brain (Goleman, 1996. p. 3-29). For our purposes here it is sufficient to understand that it is not possible for the amygdala to fully weigh up the current situation before initiating an emotional response. This means that when we 'react', we are always reacting to something that happened in our past rather than the current situation, which may be similar but significantly different.

Let us examine for a moment our behaviour when we are in the grip of an 'emotional hijacking'. As we saw earlier, in the paragraph on cognitive behaviourism, it is possible for our thoughts to influence our feelings. This is because the amygdala appears to be unable to distinguish a real event from an imaginary one. We experience an emotional response when we watch movies, or reminisce about distressing events. We become distressed again and can even trigger anxiety, because the amygdala has initiated an emotional response as though we were in the situation for real. This is also the mechanism behind what Goleman (1996) terms depressogenic thinking: habitual negative thinking that triggers fear, anxiety and depression, and the mechanism responsible for Post Traumatic Stress Disorder

(PTSD). The PTSD sufferer experiences repetitions of the traumatic event, continual 'playbacks' which trigger an emotional response from the amygdala, so they are permanently in a state of emotional arousal which they are unable to 'switch off'.

We experience the same mechanism, albeit to a lesser degree, when we are worried or when we have had a particularly busy day and are unable to switch off. When we 'replay' events in our mind, our bodies are responding as though we are still in the situation. For healthcare professionals, this might mean replaying an emergency situation which we experienced that day, and reviewing our actions. Such thoughts are capable of stimulating an emotional response and our bodies can be generating as much adrenaline as though we were still in the situation, which is why we sometimes experience 'anxiety' symptoms (palpitations, sweating, tremors), even though we are at home and the real situation is over.

THE MENTAL SPIN-CYCLE

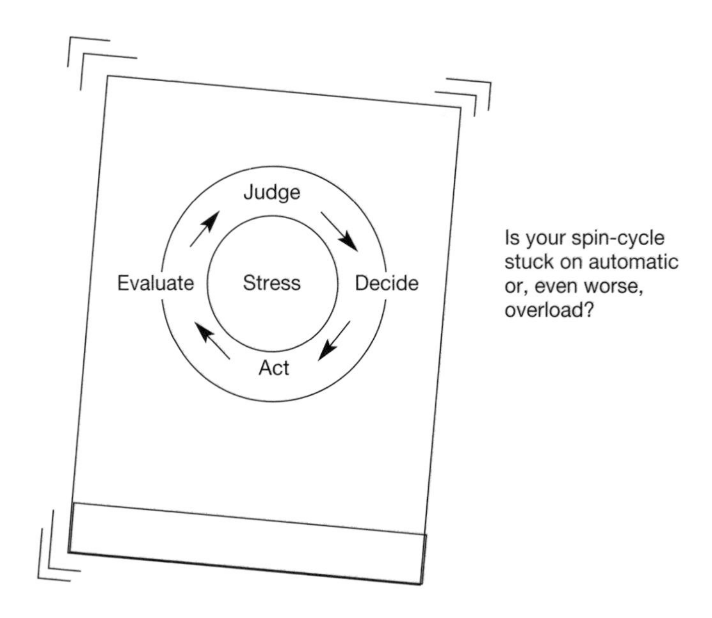

Figure 2.3 The mental spin-cycle

As healthcare practitioners, our strength often lies in our ability to judge a situation accurately, arrive at a quick decision, take appropriate action and evaluate it, which brings us back to making another judgement. This is a skill, and a valuable strength, yet it becomes problematic when we lose our conscious control over the process. I refer to this as the mental spin-cycle. Imagine a washing machine that has become stuck on 'automatic' or even on overload. Similarly we can become stuck in a continual cycle of judging> deciding> acting>evaluating, then judging – and the whole cycle repeats itself (see Figure 2.3).

Even when our clinical skills are not required, such as in our personal lives, and in our dealings with friends and colleagues, we can find ourselves continually judging, diagnosing, analysing, criticising and blaming. Consider how much energy this takes up. No wonder we find it difficult to switch off and relax.

EXERCISE

For the next week, do not judge anybody, including yourself, or anything that happens. Record what you notice about yourself in your coaching journal. Of course, you may exercise your clinical judgement as usual but pay particular attention to situations when you may be exercising your judgement when it is uninvited, inappropriate and uncalled for. Just notice. Remember, part of this exercise is to not judge yourself either!

(I am keen to hear your experience of this exercise. If you are willing, please e-mail your feedback to ruth@dreamcoach.co.uk)

The key to regaining control of this mechanism, so that we can utilise our judgement when we choose to, yet not become dominated by it when we want to switch off, is to practice being a calm observer of ourselves. If we can experience an event, or thoughts of an event, and stay relaxed, our amygdala finally learns that we are not in danger. The coaching process encourages us to become skilled at being a calm, objective observer of ourselves and creates a relaxed environment in which we feel safe and can regain control of our 'spin-cycle' switch.

We learn not to react by re-conditioning our amygdala. In situations where our amygdala has learned to trigger an emotional response we can, if we experience enough similar situations where we can remain calm and relaxed, learn to not react. According to Goleman (1996) this has been demonstrated in people suffering from PTSD which, until recently, was considered to be untreatable. As mentioned earlier, the PTSD sufferer experiences a permanent state of emotional arousal so they experience a continuous mild 'fear: fight or flight' state. It does not require much stimulus to trigger a full response, which explains their emotional hypersensitivity and 'exaggerated startle response'. They over-react to stimuli and, rather than calming down relatively quickly, they remain in a prolonged state of emotional arousal in which they may experience anxiety, tachycardia, palpitations, sweating and difficulty breathing. This is also the mechanism of a panic attack or anxiety state. When the brain is re-conditioned, we learn not to produce this emotional reaction. In the treatment of emotional trauma sufferers three stages have been identified which are essential to emotional re-learning:

1. *attaining a sense of safety;*
2. *remembering the details of the trauma to mourn the loss it has brought, and*
3. *re-establishing a normal life.*

(Herman, 1992)

Coaches have a repertoire of skills and techniques which are highly effective in working with coachees on raising their EQ, including gaining control over their thoughts and emotions. These are outlined in more detail in Chapter 3 and include techniques such as breathing, relaxation and visualisation within the safe environment provided by the coaching session. These techniques have been used effectively, within the context of a series of coaching sessions, to reduce fear and anxiety in nursing staff who have been victims of workplace bullying (Hadikin, 2002).

It has been noted that workplace bullying is extremely traumatic for the person who is targeted and can even lead to PTSD (Hadikin and O'Driscoll, 2000). Coaching can encompass the three essential criteria necessary to effect the emotional re-learning as described by Herman (1992):

1 *The coaching session, and the coach's personal style, can create a sense of safety.*

2 *Journalling, reflection and talking with the coach afford the opportunity to 'mourn' the trauma (in this case, the effects of bullying).*

3 *Various coaching techniques can be used which enable the coachee to re-establish a normal life.*

Following coaching, targets of workplace bullying have reported increased confidence, feeling relaxed at work, an improved working relationship with the bully and a cessation of bullying behaviour (Hadikin, 2002). This has obvious implications for our relationships with each other and our whole working environment. Coaching has the potential to improve matters significantly throughout the organisation, by increasing the overall level of EQ.

IMPROVING OUR RELATIONSHIPS AT WORK

Bullying, harassment, mobbing, horizontal violence and intimidation are examples of low EQ. Such behaviour is an outmoded, ineffective and expensive way to communicate. The cost of compensation payments for workplace bullying alone have been noted at over £200,000 (Hadikin and O'Driscoll, 2000). When the human species still lived in small tribal communities of less than 150 people, with no transport, media or telecommunications, such behaviour served as an effective, if somewhat brutal, form of social control. As a species, we are evolving into a global community. We are collectively maturing and outgrowing this immature behaviour. The demands of our modern age, our global society, with its ability to connect across regions, nations, class, creed and culture, means we need to develop a highly advanced way to communicate with each other, and fast. Coaching is a highly advanced form of communication. In future, coaching may not only be a tool used by professionals but a communication style available to us all. Where any such behaviours are present in a workplace, effective coaching can improve matters significantly by increasing the level of EQ.

POLARISED RELATIONSHIPS

The bully-victim dyad is an example of a polarised relationship. In polarised relationships, one person adopts an extreme behaviour pattern while the other person adopts an equally extreme 'opposite' behaviour pattern. Under stress, our behaviour patterns become more extreme and exaggerated and provoke an extreme opposite response in the other person. An example could be over-responding or over-functioning. If one person in a relationship has a tendency to over-respond in stressful situations, to take charge and organise others, the other person in this relationship may increasingly under-respond, lose touch with their own competence and take a passive role. According to Lerner (1989) the two people then get locked into a circular 'dance' which is self-perpetuating and can become 'stuck'. In other words, this becomes an entrenched behaviour pattern and might feel 'normal' for the people involved in this relationship. Since the behaviours are dependent on one another, each relies on the other to perpetuate their own behaviour, neither seems able to alter their behaviour pattern while in this relationship. In this instance, the two people in the relationship are dependent on each other in order to enable them to maintain this role. The over-responder depends on the under-responder's passivity, which enables them to continue over-functioning. The under-responder depends on the over-responder to take all the responsibility, enabling them to continue under-functioning and avoiding any responsibility (Bowen, 1978).

The underlying factor is our natural tendency to fall into a familiar pattern when under stress. We may have learned this pattern in childhood and possibly it is a pattern that serves us in some way in our family context. We can identify with elements of over-functioning and under-functioning in our existing relationships, both at home and at work. We may also note that these are not fixed character traits and that we may under-function in one relationship and/or role and find ourselves over-functioning in another.

Through working with a coach, we are able to obtain some relief from the intensity of relationships, both in our family system and our workplace, and move into a temporary feeling of objectivity within the coaching session. Calming ourselves and becoming objective is essential for us to be able to observe our own behaviour patterns in our key relationships, including those with our colleagues, developing our self-awareness, re-conditioning our emotional responses and raising our EQ.

THE CALM, OBJECTIVE, OBSERVER OF SELF

As mentioned earlier, the coach is not a therapist, and coaching is not essentially a therapeutic role. Neither is the coach in this context acting in the role of a relationship therapist but rather a facilitator of our growth so that we become, in essence, our own best expert on how we behave in our relationships. Using the coaching session to develop the role of self-observer enables us to step outside of our own situation and temporarily gain the calmness and objectivity required to think clearly. Goleman (1996) emphasises the importance of attaining a state of calmness, or relaxation, to enable the emotional brain (the amygdala) to 'switch off'. This is essential to enable our cortex (thinking brain) to function effectively. Consider how difficult it is to think clearly when we are emotionally aroused. Being calm simply enables us to think.

EXERCISE

Imagine a tiny 'Tom Thumb-sized' version of yourself, that you could hold in your hand. Use this technique to imagine looking down on yourself. Observe yourself in different relationships and various situations. It is important that you undertake this exercise without judgement of yourself. Simply notice. Notice your feelings and your reactions. Notice if you experience any judgement, and go easy on yourself. Let go of the judgement.

(I am keen to hear your experience of this exercise. If you are willing, please e-mail your feedback to ruth@dreamcoach.co.uk)

It is extremely difficult to be calm and objective when you are emotionally involved. It takes time and practice. I recommend you try the above exercise and write your observations in your coaching journal. I am not suggesting it is always wrong to make judgements. We all make judgements. It is in our nature to do so and it is often necessary to do so. As mentioned earlier, exercising our clinical judgement is an essential part of our role, which can save lives. Sometimes exercising judgement will even save our own life. Yet there are many situations in life when it really does not serve us to do so. If we judge ourselves harshly during the above exercise it increases negative thought, may reinforce negative core beliefs, and reduce our self-esteem.

When we observe ourselves without judgement, and are courageous and willing enough to observe our own patterns and those of others, we discover that we are able to remain calm enough to think clearly. This affords us the opportunity to identify several alternatives which may lie before us, evaluate the consequences of each, and choose different options for ourselves in future.

this work [on our Selves] allows us to move toward a more balanced and authentic self. It is our best insurance policy against continuing polarized relationships with new people in our lives and passing the pattern down the generations.

(Lerner, 1989. p.112.)

CHOICE AND CONTROL

The coaching philosophy emphasises that we always have choices, even though we are unaware of them at times. Being emotionally aroused clouds our thinking so that we are less able to recognise the choices we do have. Attaining a state of calm objectivity clears our thinking so that the full range of possibilities opens up before us. Behaviour and action that may have appeared to be beyond our control suddenly becomes under our control. When we realise that we have choice, it gives us the power to make different choices and experience different outcomes.

When we see a clear distinction between a choice and our nature, or temperament, it becomes much easier to separate a person from their actions. It makes it much easier for us to have unconditional positive regard. We can see much more clearly that making an unwise or 'bad' choice does not necessarily make someone a 'bad' person. Including ourselves. We can feel better about ourselves and those times in our lives when we have made poor choices. It makes it OK for us to say to ourselves: 'I am a good person, I just did some bad stuff.' This then gives us permission to change our behaviour and make 'good' choices. If we choose to.

Whether we are 'good' or 'bad' is not the issue. What matters is how we feel and, more importantly, whether we feel in control. If we have a core belief that we will do 'bad' things because we ARE 'bad' and we just cannot help it, we do not have a degree of self-efficacy. We do not possess the power to change. Acknowledging that we have a choice gives us this power. If we believe that we are basically someone who is not 'bad', but has simply made some 'bad' choices, this gives us the option of making different choices. Having choice puts us in control, and we always have a choice. If we *feel* in control of what happens to us, we *are* in control. We are empowered.

ATTRIBUTION THEORY

Heider (1958) described how we attribute motives to behaviour we observe. We make an assumption about why people, including ourselves, behave like we do. There is a self-serving bias in attribution, in that we attribute our 'good' behaviour to internal causes, within our control, yet we attribute our 'bad' behaviour to external causes, outside our control. If we help an elderly person to carry their shopping it is because we are choosing to be kind. It is a choice within our control. If we fall down drunk and fail to show up for our best friend's wedding it is because we are sick. We cannot help it, alcoholism is outside our control. Davies (1992) applies attribution theory to his work on addiction. In his view, addiction is not an illness over which we have no control, but rather a choice that we can decide to participate in or not. By emphasising choice he empowers addicts to take control of their own lives and challenges the belief that they are in the grip of an 'illness' which is beyond their control.

Davies (1992) notes how addicts may feel that they have lost their willpower and capacity for personal decision-making, yet they choose drugs because they want to and because they see no good reason for giving them up. Addictive behaviour is therefore a personal choice. Davies describes addiction as a form of learned helplessness that encourages passivity and irresponsibility.

The following is an example of coaching a coachee who drinks heavily. I want to re-emphasise that coaching is not intended as any kind of therapy and to draw your attention to the coaching dialogue in which the coach challenges the coachee's underlying assumption that she has no control by stating and re-stating that she does, in fact, have a choice.

Coaching Case Study

Jo came to me as a private coaching client. She is a healthcare manager who is on sick leave with stress-related illness. She drinks heavily, as do many of us when we are under stress. She experiences anxiety and panic attacks. She is also seeing a psychotherapist.

Jo: I'm not doing well with not drinking. I had a few again last night.

Coach: That's OK. You had a choice and you chose to drink. Try to avoid negative judgement if you can, Jo. It was simply a choice.

Jo: Yes, but I've been trying to give up and now I'm back to square one.

Coach: We're never back at square one, it's not possible. With every step, every day, we learn something new. What do you know now that you didn't know yesterday?

Jo: I feel rotten!

Coach: OK, good answer. You had a drink and you feel rotten.

Jo: Yes. I don't know why I do it when I feel so bad. I don't want to drink.

Coach: What is the truth, Jo?

Jo: Pardon?

Coach: Is it true that you don't want to drink?

Jo: Yes!

Coach: I hear that, in this moment, you feel rotten and you really don't want to drink; however I believe that last night you did want to drink, which is why you drank!

Jo: I suppose I did.

Coach: And that's OK too. Just notice that you had a choice and you chose to drink.

Jo: But it's not OK because I don't want to live like this.

Coach: Good. So choose differently.

Jo: It's so hard though. I get tempted, and then I get stressed out and I think 'to hell with it!' and I drink.

Coach: How does it serve you?

Jo: It makes me feel better.

Coach: Yes it does! How do you feel when you are stressed out?

Jo: I get anxious, my hands shake, I can't breathe... I have knots in my stomach... I feel terrible...

Coach: And having a drink takes all that away as quick as a flash?

Jo: Almost, yes. I feel great after just one drink!

Coach: It seems to me like you've found a quick and easy way to relieve your anxiety.

Jo: Yes, I have but...

Coach: But what?

Jo: ...it's not healthy, I worry about my liver and my reputation – I don't want to be a drunk.

Coach: Great!

Jo: Great?

Coach: Yes, it's great that you know that about yourself. You want to relieve your anxiety and you don't want to damage your health. You have found a quick way to relieve your anxiety through drinking. The disadvantage is that it is damaging your health in the long-term. You want to be healthy. You drink to feel better. Drinking is damaging you. No wonder you feel so rotten: your actions are so out of accord with your beliefs and integrity. What would be some ways to relieve your anxiety, that would feel more in integrity for you?

Jo: Going running I suppose...

Coach: Yes, you are an excellent runner Jo, (the coach is aware that Jo was well placed in the London marathon) and exercise is great for lowering stress. What else?

Jo: Doing relaxation exercises...

Coach: Another good one, yes. What else?

Jo: Gardening... walking... meditation...

Coach: I love it! Yes, they are all superb. So, can you see how many choices you have now?

Jo: Yes, but it's still quicker to drink.

Coach: Yes it is. And that will always be your choice: 'Do I have this drink, go for a quick fix, and then feel out of integrity, or do I make a healthier choice, feel better more slowly, and feel better about myself?' It's your choice.

Throughout the coaching session (of which the above dialogue is but a small part) I continue to emphasise that Jo has choices and to help her see what they are. Yet at the same time I am not suggesting there is a quick fix available, or that any of this will be easy. There is compassion, empathy and realism. Yes, drinking is a fast way to relieve anxiety and whether it is the method of choice is up to Jo. It is her choice. It is her responsibility. It is my role as coach to remind her of this and to show her where she has choice and power. This puts her in control.

MOMENTUM

This might be a good time to mention that coaching is most effective through regular coaching sessions. One off 'hit and run' sessions can prove very effective as brainstorming sessions, but without the request for action and regular feedback it can hardly be considered coaching in a true sense. Checking in with our coach at regular periods, in person, by telephone and/or e-mail, is essential to keep us focused on our goals, develop our EQ and maintain momentum. This momentum is what keeps the coachee making steady progress toward their goals. Without the ongoing support afforded by regular coaching we will, after time, resort to our familiar behaviour.

ACTION LEARNING

The coaching call is only the beginning. The real learning takes place between coaching sessions as we take action, make changes in our lives, then reflect and learn from those actions which are more or less successful for us. As we observe ourselves and note our observations there is an element of reflective learning. Through reflection, we observe our own part in creating or perpetuating the circumstances we are in. We notice where we give away our power to others, how circumstances can change, and what we can do. We begin to recognise where we have choices. We experiment. We might agree to a request or action suggested by the coach. Then we evaluate our action or behaviour to discern whether it feels appropriate for us to continue. Coaching encourages reflection, action-learning and enhances experiential learning. We develop emotional maturity as we experience ourselves uniquely by observing our Selves living our own lives.

3

Coaching skills, tools, terms and techniques

Far beyond ideas of right-doing and wrong-doing
There is a field.
I'll meet you there.

Rumi

Coaching is eclectic and draws upon many tools and techniques to fulfil its aim of facilitating personal and organisational growth. This chapter outlines some of the skills, tools, techniques, approaches and terminology used in coaching. This list is by no means exhaustive. Coaching is essentially a creative art, and the coach is free to literally make it up as she goes along, in the respect that she creates new tools, metaphors and techniques as she 'dances' with each unique client. Coaches may use some or all of the methods listed here, and some may use methods which are not listed here. Many of these skills and techniques are also used in other professions and may well be familiar to you if you already use them in your practice or indeed if you have experience of being coached.

As implied by the term 'coaching', much of the influence has come from the USA and many coaching terms derive from American-English and may seem unusual to readers in the UK. In this chapter, common coaching terms are explained in alphabetical order so, in effect, it also acts as a glossary for some of the unusual language we may stumble across as we examine the influence of, and potential for, coaching in healthcare.

ACCOUNTABILITY

As distinct from professional accountability, literally 'holding to account' is a key element of any coaching relationship. Holding the client to account hallmarks the difference between a coaching relationship and many other kinds of professional relationships, such as counselling. The language the coach uses is usually quite specific. For example:

Are you willing to try that?

When will you do it, John?

How will I know?

It is this level of accountability that encourages the coachee to take action sooner, rather than later, and to follow-through on their ideas and plans. Sharing our commitment with another has a powerful psychological effect. It somehow deepens the commitment so we are more likely to honour it. In addition to the commitment to ourselves, there is something about sharing our plans with another person that makes us more likely to stick to them.

For example, imagine we tell ourselves we will give up sugar. Then one hour into the first day someone offers us a piece of chocolate. It is so easy to simply eat the chocolate and tell ourselves we can begin again tomorrow. If we have told someone of our plans, and we know they will follow up, it makes us think twice before breaking our own commitment to ourselves.

ACKNOWLEDGING

Coachees often commit to making dramatic changes in themselves and may also be overcoming long-standing challenges. Acknowledgement from the coach of their effort, commitment, determination, courage, gifts and talents is a wonderfully empowering and motivating experience. It is necessary for our continued growth and development. Though it is difficult to explain precisely why acknowledgement is so effective in spurring us on, it is easy to see how disillusioned we become when we do not receive any acknowledgement of our efforts. The complaint I have probably heard most often from healthcare professionals is that they do not feel acknowledged in their work. When we are acknowledged we feel affirmed and validated. We feel appreciated.

ACTING 'AS IF'

This is not so much a coaching skill as a technique that the coach may request the coachee to employ. Acting 'as if' refers to the ability to act as if we are already in the position we desire to be in. This means adopting the appropriate behaviour patterns and allowing ourselves the experience of 'playing' with the role. Even though we may only be role-playing or pretending, we may experience how we would feel in the role. It is in effect a rehearsal and an important part of learning necessary skills. It can be used effectively in conjunction with visualisation (below).

It differs from role play in that we do not set aside a separate time and play out the role with someone who has agreed to role play. Rather like a method actor preparing for a role, we try to adjust ourselves mentally, to connect with our feelings, and try to live out our day 'acting as if' we are the person we wish to become.

ACTION PLANNING

The coaching focus is always on taking action. Preferably effective action. Coaching focuses on doing what works and on letting go of what does not work. During most coaching sessions the coach will request some action from the coachee. This may sound as though the coach is creating more work but sometimes the action required might be to actually do less.

Any action taken is always evaluated for effectiveness. The coachee is encouraged to review their action for effectiveness and give feedback. Then the coach may request another action or a modified version of the first action. There is sometimes an element of trial and error until coachee and coach discover the most effective way forward. There is also scope for action learning and experiential learning as the coachee reviews the effects and consequences of any action taken and reflects on their experience.

Action can be planned over the long term, as incremental stages within an overall strategy, or may be in the form of a daily action list, or may just be a one-off request from the coach. Daily action lists are always goal-specific. The coach's aim in requesting action is to keep the coachee making steady progress towards their goals.

ARTICULATING TRUTH

What is really going on? What is true for the coachee in this situation? What is true for the coach? Articulating truth is a skill that some of us are not comfortable with at first. We know that 'truth' is subjective. It is not absolute and depends on our perspective yet articulating 'truth' is an essential part of coaching. It builds trust and helps the coachee to accept the present reality. When the coachee is willing to accept the reality of their situation they are in a position to start planning how they want to change their reality. Until they accept reality they will not be able to change.

Acceptance of the present reality, no matter how uncomfortable we may be with it, is the only place from which we can move forward. The inquiry process and challenging our thoughts (see Chapter 2) lead us to acceptance. Only when we know where we are can we plan how to move on from this place. If we want to go to Edinburgh and we do not know whether we are in Dover, Dublin or Dieppe how can we plan our route?

So how do we define 'truth'? The truth is whatever is true for us in that moment. With hindsight and/or more information our opinion may change, but for the purpose of the coaching session, the truth for us is how we see it there and then. The truth for the coachee is how they see it.

It is difficult to strike a balance between unconditional positive regard (see 'make the coachee right' below) and challenging a coachee who is not facing up to something. It is an important part of the coaching relationship to acknowledge the reality of a situation. As we become masterful in our coaching skills we learn to walk the fine line by confronting a coachee with reality and delivering the message in a compassionate way. A master coach learns to 'listen between the lines'. That is, to listen for what the client is not saying as well as what they are. This is where it is important for a coach to have an opinion and to be willing to share it.

As an example, here is an extract from a coaching dialogue with a coachee who is anxious about an impending redundancy:

Coach: In this present moment you are safe.

Coachee: I'm not safe. I might lose my house and I might lose my job, so there are all these things that might happen and I'm not safe.

Coach: I hear that you don't feel safe right now. However the reality is that, in this moment, you haven't lost your job or your house. I'm not saying it won't happen in the future but in this present moment, as we speak, it isn't happening. You are safe.

In the above example the coach makes the coachee 'right' by acknowledging that she does not feel safe while at the same time pointing out the reality that, in this moment, she actually is safe because the event which she is afraid may happen has not happened. We may think it will happen, or it could happen, but if we are to articulate truth in this instance the reality is that it has not happened.

Acceptance of reality does not mean resignation, submission or giving up. It does not mean we have to like it and it does not mean we cannot change it but we do have to accept it if we are to be able to move on.

ASKING PERMISSION

Asking permission brings clarity and effectiveness to our communication. An effective coach always asks permission before sharing intuitions, before giving fieldwork, before requesting and before playing. Examples include:

May I share with you my hunch around this?

May I make a request of you?

May I suggest a piece of fieldwork?

Are you willing to play a game here?

Would you like some role play on this?

'BEING WITH' THE COACHEE

Sometimes it is enough to simply be with the coachee. Sometimes all a coachee wants from a coaching session is to be with somebody who cares. Being able to be with coachees without speaking, being comfortable with silence and being comfortable with our coachee's emotions, whatever they may be, is a skill that coaches can develop. This may involve active listening or not. It may simply involve sitting with somebody.

Being with people is a skill which is undervalued in our fast-paced society. How many of us are comfortable to sit with a dying friend or relative? Or to sit with a friend in labour? Sometimes our coachees, for whatever reason, feel alone. It may be that they are initiating dramatic changes in their lives and feel that no one understands or agrees with them. They may be creating something new and do not have anyone in their support network who grasps the concept yet. Whatever the reason, sometimes they just need someone on their side to simply be with them. They might just need somebody in their corner. Being with a coachee does not mean we are doing nothing. It takes our full attention and presence. It is not a case of sitting there and daydreaming about what we are going to have for dinner this evening, or planning our next holiday. When we are being with a coachee our full attention is on them. 100% in the moment. We are fully present.

BRAINSTORMING

Brainstorming is a common reason why people use a coach. During a typical brainstorming session both coach and coachee will take turns thinking of ideas and options and the result will be to generate much more information than either would have thought of alone. The point of a brainstorming session is to generate ideas and/or information. In setting up the brainstorming session the coach will usually ask permission: 'Would you like to brainstorm around this?'

The coach might begin by suggesting an idea or two, then invite the coachee to join in with their ideas, and eventually they take turns until they have exhausted all their ideas. During the brainstorming it helps to just generate idea after idea and not evaluate them at this stage. Some ideas might sound impossible, far-fetched or just plain silly, but brainstorming is a creative process and the idea is to let it flow, allow our creativity to gather momentum and generate new material. If we evaluate ideas at this stage it impedes the flow, stifles the generation of new ideas and halts the creative process. It is therefore important not to judge our ideas but to continue in spite of any apparent 'silliness'.

CHALLENGING

Setting a challenge is how a coach stretches a coachee beyond their perceived ability. We become creatures of habit so easily. Last year, when I began swimming regularly, I could only swim 14 lengths. Every couple of months I increased this by challenging myself to swim further than I believed I could. Once I became comfortable with 30 lengths (meaning I could swim 30 easily) I challenged myself to swim 32. Where our coachees appear to have levelled off, and we know they can achieve more, we can challenge them to. An example might be: 'I challenge you to walk for 30 minutes every day.' They may agree, or may respond with a counter-offer: 'I'll do 20.'

Setting a challenge is how we initiate a new phase of growth and encourage coachees to reach beyond, and exceed, their own limitations. When we begin coaching, as coachees, we are often in our own 'comfort zone'. We may know where we want to make changes in our lives but, for the moment, we are comfortable with what we have, even if it is not what we want, because it is familiar. Accepting a challenge means moving out of the familiar and into the unknown. This is scary territory: anything can happen. It may not be comfortable but it can be exciting and very stimulating. We can become bored with the familiar. Once we have become accustomed to our 'new' level of expertise it will very soon become familiar to us and may well become another comfort zone unless we challenge ourselves to stretch a little further. By continually monitoring ourselves in terms of boredom and challenge we can manage to stay in a state of flow (see Chapter 2).

It is important at this point to mention another meaning for the term 'challenging' which is to dispute something. This is linked to articulating the truth (above) and is a skill which is a valuable part of a coaching relationship. In this sense a coach will challenge a coachee who appears out of touch with the reality of a situation. A coach may also challenge negative thoughts and core beliefs by asking: 'Is that true?' (see Chapter 2).

CHAMPIONING

This is where we have higher expectations of the coachee than the coachee does of herself, and we express them. Expressing our high expectations of our coachees encourages them to rise to the occasion. The coach can often see potential in a coachee that the coachee herself cannot. In coaching we expect them to exceed their self-imposed limitations simply because that is what humans are capable of. We exceed our own limitations all the time and constantly amaze ourselves. Championing helps us to overcome temporary lows and self-doubt. When our coach still believes in us, even when we lose our self-belief, we begin to think: 'If my coach believes I can do it, maybe I can.' We know our own potential. We just lose sight of it sometimes. Having a coach to remind us is empowering, affirming, validating, inspiring and motivating. We feel spurred on. Restoring our self-belief in this way re-connects us with our potential and our sense of self: our sense of who we really are.

CHARGE NEUTRAL

Charge neutral means speaking in a neutral tone of voice without an emotional charge. This technique is sometimes employed by coaches during coaching sessions, especially when challenging a coachee. If we challenge our coachees with an emotional overtone in our voice it may be received as threatening or intimidating. When we feel threatened we do not listen; rather, we prepare our defence. When we challenge a coachee we deliver the message directly, to ensure we are heard, and we let them know we feel compassion by adopting a charge neutral tone. (See 'the edge' below.)

CLARIFYING

It is important that we understand precisely what the coachee means. During the coaching session we stop them periodically to gain clarification and check we have understood their meaning correctly. We do this in several ways. We might repeat exactly what the coachee just said (mirroring) or paraphrase (reporting back in our own words) what we understood them to mean. To introduce to the coachee that this is what we are doing we may simply ask: 'Have I understood that correctly?' or 'Let me check that I have understood you, Tom, do you mean...?'

In checking for clarity not only do we, as coaches, gain clarity but so does the coachee. In listening to our version of what they said they have the opportunity to clarify their meaning. This leads to greater clarity for the coachee as well as the coach.

CLEAN SWEEP

Part of the coach's role is to help the coachee to create a clear pathway to achieving their goal. This means looking at whatever is blocking or obstructing them. Many coaches will begin by 'clearing the decks' or 'making a clean sweep'. This involves requesting the coachee to review every aspect of their life including relationships, finances, work, environment and health to identify where they invest most of their time, attention and energy, and make changes in many or all of these areas to effect a 'clean sweep'.

Many of us invest much of our time and energy in activities which we do not enjoy and have no desire to do. A review of this nature can help us to become aware of just how much time and energy we are spending in such areas, which can explain why we have little time or energy left over to invest in our goals and plans. It can also help us to identify what areas we can change to free up some time and energy to invest elsewhere. Looking at how we manage all these areas of our lives can be very illuminating. In learning to manage some areas differently, by making different choices and learning how to do certain things differently, we may be able to free up much more time and energy than we imagined. Have you ever stopped and wondered: 'How do other people manage to do all this and still have time left over to play?'

By undertaking a systematic review of where your time and energy is going, you may learn how others do manage and still have time left over to spend on themselves.

To help us understand how a coach may approach this, let us use the area of finances as an example. The first step is the review, or 'reality check'. As mentioned earlier, we cannot choose a route to our destination without knowing our starting point, or point of reference. The coach would request the coachee make a thorough review of their financial position including what their income and expenditure is, whether they draw up and live within a budget, how much they owe and how much they save.

The next step is to identify the destination. This would mean exploring the coachee's goals in relation to their finances. If they are aiming for financial security, what does that mean to them? The coach would encourage them to be as specific as possible in defining their goal, or destination. Then coach and coachee together can identify the gap between where the coachee is now, in terms of their finances, and where they want to be. The next step is to co-create a strategy for how they are going to get there. Using some of the coaching skills and techniques mentioned here the coach may enable the coachee to clear any outstanding debt, improve their money management skills and put structures in place to ensure their money continues to grow and remain stable. This cannot mean a one-off effort and then ignoring the financial situation again. A money management system might mean using computer software to keep a weekly, monthly and annual account of income and expenses, calculating a personal budget, then staying within it. A coach will always encourage the coachee to create a permanent solution to prevent problems appearing in future. This would mean that the coachee learns new habits, new ways of habitually and regularly monitoring their financial picture. It may also mean overcoming a fear of managing money that many of us have.

The coaching process is not only demonstrated in a 'clean sweep'. The process is the same in any of the above-mentioned 'life' areas. This is an opportune moment to include a brief overview of the coaching process, which may help to place many of these coaching skills and techniques in context:

1. *The reference point*
   The coach guides the coachee towards taking a reality check or clean sweep. This is a review of the current reality which requires the coachee to be honest with themselves. What is the present reality?

2. *The goal or destination*
   Where does the coachee want to be, what is the destination?

3. *The gap*
   What is the difference between where the coachee is now and where they want to be? Is the goal realistic and feasible?

4. *The strategy*
   Identifying what needs to be done, co-creating a method and putting structure in place to enable the client to bridge the gap.

5. *Overcoming obstacles*
   What is holding the coachee back? Do they have fears and/or reservations about moving towards their goal? Are they overwhelmed by other demands and commitments which utilise their time and energy? Do they need to free up some time and energy from elsewhere to devote to this project? Where do they experience resistance?

6. *Being there*
   The coach is there with ongoing support to provide the inspiration, focus and motivation which enables the coachee to keep taking the steps along the path toward their goal and to keep their structures in place.

CO-CREATING

As mentioned earlier, coaching is a partnership between equals in which coach and coachee have equal responsibility for co-creating the results. We are co-creators of the coaching relationship and co-creators of their strategy and/or action plan. The coach is willing to share fully her ideas, creativity and contributions. The coachee participates fully and does not rely on the coach to come up with all the answers. In this way both are equally responsible for creating the results.

COMMITMENT

Commitment is a vital aspect of successful coaching. When we enter the coaching relationship we make a personal commitment to ourselves and to achieving our goals. We commit ourselves to whatever steps are necessary to make them a reality. As coaches we commit to being there for our coachees and to offering the unconditional positive regard which nurtures the coaching relationship. Both coach and coachee are fully committed to the coaching relationship.

The coaching relationship is the context within which the essential synergy is created, nurtured and maintained. This cannot exist without mutual commitment. Without mutual commitment the coaching will be ineffective.

CONFIDENTIALITY

Confidentiality is essential for the coaching relationship to work. For the duration of the coaching relationship the coach has access to sensitive information about the coachee's life and business affairs. Coaching cannot work without trust, and trust cannot be built without a confidentiality agreement which is strictly enforced. Professional coaches often make this explicit in a written coaching agreement.

CREATING TRUST

Trust is essential for the coaching relationship to work. How trust develops depends on the coach and the coachee. Trust develops through a combination of the coach's personal style and skill and how well they are 'matched' with the coachee. Often, in choosing a coach, the coachee will choose someone with similar standards of integrity, personal standards and confidentiality.

DANCING

Every relationship is a 'dance' in the sense that the people involved are partners moving forward in tandem, working together, synchronised. At the beginning of a coaching session we begin from 'where the coachee is'. This might mean matching their mood and tone of voice. Then the 'dance' begins. As coaches become increasingly proficient in their own emotional and relationship skills they become better 'dancers' with their coachees.

DETACHMENT FROM THE OUTCOME

The coaching relationship is co-created for the purpose of advancing the coachee. The focus of every coaching relationship is therefore always the coachee's agenda. This means the coach remains detached from the outcome. For example, a coachee might decide on working towards a course of study, such as a degree programme, and undertake study to qualify, such as an access course or further education. Following this the coachee might change their mind and not apply for the degree course after all. The coach's role is to help the coachee clarify their path and make the right choice for them, rather than continue 'pushing' the coachee to take the degree course. It is precisely this perception of 'pushiness' that is avoided by detaching from the outcome. If we have no attachment to our coachee's course of action we will continue to nurture their growth without stifling them. The coachee will then feel free to flow in any direction they choose.

This is also the case with in-house coaching, where the coach may be the coachee's manager, and there are organisational objectives which must be met. During the coaching session, the coach manager learns to temporarily let go of organisational objectives and switch focus to the coachee's personal development. The specific challenges of the coach manager are discussed in greater depth in Chapter 6. Attachment can limit coaches (including managers) in a real sense. If your success is dependent upon your coachee's performance then you are attached to the outcome. You will be 'pushy' in your coaching style, you will 'need' the result too much, and your coaching will be ineffective.

Effective coaching occurs where the coach has no attachment whatsoever to the coachee's outcome.

EMPOWERING

Empowering in itself is not a tangible skill but rather the result produced by a combination of skills such as validating, affirming, acknowledging, creating trust, identifying choice and holding our coachees in unconditional positive regard.

We are never powerless, yet we often may feel so. For some reason we seem unable to exercise the power we have. We feel disempowered. In *The Bullying Culture* (Hadikin and O'Driscoll, 2000) we noted how disempowered many midwives felt and yet, to their clients, midwives were in positions of tremendous power. What an astonishing difference in perception, that a group of people who appear to have enormous power can feel so disempowered. It is for this reason that I am not particularly enamoured of the term 'empowerment'. It implies we have no power, whereas in fact we have power that we do not realise we have. Coaching helps us to recognise where we do have choices and, in exercising them, we do have power.

A coach 'empowers' us by helping to identify where we have

choice and control and to recognise how we disempower ourselves through behaviour that effectively gives our power over to others. As coaches we may even enquire of a coachee: 'Where do you give up your power?'

GIVING FIELDWORK

For coaching to be effective it is essential to move the coachee forward towards their stated goal. If this is not happening it is not coaching. Setting fieldwork, making requests and challenging are the coach's way of ensuring the coachee commits to action that will move them forward.

GOAL-SETTING AND BOOK-ENDING

Goals can be immediate, short-term, medium-term or long-term. They can be linked directly to our vision and strategy or may be smaller goals to achieve a specific result. Goals, however large or small, should always be SMART (see Chapter 2).

Book-ending is a term sometimes used in coaching to describe where an immediate, specific request is combined with immediate follow-up and feedback to achieve a goal quickly. The request and follow-up are 'book-ends' to the goal. For example:

Coach: I request you make that phone call now, and call me right back when you've done it. Are you willing to do that, John?

Coachee: Yes.

Coach: Great, go and make that call then and I'll await your return call.

John hangs up and makes his call. Then he calls the coach back.

Coach: Hi John, how did it go?

The 'book-ends' of the request at one end, with the feedback and accountability at the other, support the action in the moment. This is useful to achieve a quick success which nurtures the coachee's self-belief and especially useful in overcoming fear.

HOLDING THE COACHEE'S AGENDA

During the initial coaching session, the focus of coaching is agreed on. The nature and scope of the coaching is defined from the start. The coach then holds the coachee's agenda throughout future coaching sessions. This means that as the coachee becomes distracted by the various stages in the coaching process, more immediate short-term goals, overcoming obstacles and dealing with other matters in her life which demand her time and attention, the coach always holds the 'bigger picture', acts as an anchor and reminds the coachee of her overall aim.

The coachee's agenda may change and there should be enough flexibility in a coaching relationship to allow for this. This happens as people grow and develop more clarity regarding their future plans.

INQUIRY

Coaching is essentially a process of supported inquiry. The coach asks questions which encourage the coachee to use her skills, talents, resourcefulness, knowledge, creativity, strengths and wisdom to create solutions, overcome challenges, reach for higher goals and discover a greater sense of self in the process. Coaching becomes most effective when it is a process of self-inquiry. This happens as the coach asks questions that arise from genuine interest and curiosity which encourage reflection in the coachee. This style of questioning marks a distinct deviation from the information-gathering 'diagnostic' style of questions familiar to most healthcare practitioners. There is also a myth that coaching is simply about asking questions, and many inexperienced novice coaches make the mistake of simply firing one question after another at their coachees. Questioning is a skill that must be applied judiciously if the coachee is not to feel as though they are subject to some form of interrogation. One well-placed question, that encourages the coachee to reflect and inquire within, may outweigh a dozen information-gathering questions.

Many novice coaches also make the mistake of focusing too much of their attention on creating the 'great coaching question' which will inspire their coachee toward a breakthrough. Care must be taken to ensure our attention is with the coachee at all times (see 'presence', below). If our attention is on creating a great question and/or being a great coach, we are not fully with our coachees. We do better to listen attentively and 'be with' them. The questions that then arise within us, from our natural concern and curiosity, are always appropriate.

INTRUDING/TAKING CHARGE

This seems to contradict the ethos of empowering and working to the coachee's agenda, yet it is an essential part of coaching which helps keep the coachee on track. Sometimes, as coachees, we become adept at avoiding our own agendas. Have you ever managed to successfully avoid studying? Look how many strategies you can come up with as avoidance techniques. If our coachees continue in the same patterns, and respond in the same way as they always have done, their lives will not alter much. There is an axiom in coaching that goes like this: 'If you do what you've always done, you'll get what you've always got.' This means that if we want to produce different results we have to take different action. If we whisk up eggs and throw them into a frying pan we will always get an omelette. If we want a different result we must do something different with our eggs.

To make dramatic changes we must take action that is dramatically different from how we would normally approach things. This is uncomfortable, unfamiliar and may require skills that we do not yet possess. Resistance is perfectly understandable. When a coach realises that a coachee is repeating an old story, or is stuck in an old behaviour pattern or drama, it is in their best interest for the coach to interrupt and point out to them that they may need to look at things differently if they want anything to change. The skilled coach interrupts in a sensitive manner and gently returns the coachee's attention to her original agenda. The only time a coach intrudes and takes over is to bring a coachee back to her own goals in her own interest. It is never for the coach's own agenda, for an ego trip or for the benefit of 'being right'.

Interrupting is a valuable coaching skill. Projecting our own agenda onto the coachee is not.

INTUITION

What is intuition? A gut feeling? A sixth sense? An inkling about something?

It has been acknowledged by psychologists (Peck, 1990) that, although these factors are inherently difficult to examine from a scientific viewpoint, there is invariably useful information which is delivered to us through the 'unconscious' or subconscious part of our minds.

While these 'idle thoughts' usually provide us with insight into ourselves, they may also provide us with dramatic insights into others or into the world outside ourselves.

(Peck, 1990)

This is important information that cannot be overlooked on a coaching call if our aim is to facilitate the overall physical, mental, emotional and spiritual development of our coachees. My most successful coaching has been where I have shared my intuition and have encouraged my coachees to also pay attention to theirs and act upon it. I spoke with a coachee who is finally moving out after living with her boyfriend for two years. She told me:

I knew at the time it was the wrong thing to do. All my alarm bells were ringing and my gut feeling was don't do this... but it made perfect sense and I couldn't think of a logical reason not to. So I went ahead.

She suffered two years of misery before realising that, despite logic, this situation was not appropriate for her.

We live in a world where logic rules. So much so that we often feel obliged to pursue whatever seems to be the 'logical thing to do' when all our senses are screaming at us to do otherwise. Yet all our logic, reason and rationalising does not take our emotional world into account. Emotionally, we operate in a different realm and sometimes we know what is right for us when we have nothing more to go on than 'that funny feeling I get in the pit of my stomach'!

Somewhere in our desire for science to expand our knowledge we have made it unacceptable to use valuable tools if we are unable to demonstrate scientifically how they work. We do not need to understand how electricity is formed to be able to turn on the light. Of course there is room for more research in this area and one of the major stumbling blocks has been a lack of acceptable scientific methodology. Intuition, as with many intangible phenomena, is difficult to measure precisely because we cannot see it to observe it. This does not mean it does not exist.

We can still give ourselves permission to use the tool while we await the evidence to explain to us how it works. In evidence-based practice we do not require evidence of how intuition works, only evidence that it does. To gather this evidence we must first allow ourselves to use intuition intentionally before we can observe and record our results. It is up to us to collect this evidence.

INVENTION (MAKING IT UP!)

In some coaching texts this is referred to as 'Make It Up' (CoachU, 1999). If the coachee seems blocked, stuck or 'bogged down' looking for an answer, encourage them to create one by 'making it up' there and then. You might ask a question such as: 'If you had the perfect solution right now, what would it look like?'

If they say 'I don't know', suggest they make it up. What could it look like? This is great at unblocking creativity and prompting the inspiration to start flowing again. If the coachee is still blank, you can make it up. A light playful approach is essential for creativity, including thinking up creative solutions to obstacles, problems or challenges. As a coach you could begin by making something up yourself.

Coach: Hey, have you thought of __________ ?

Coachee: Wow! Will that work?

Coach: I don't know, I just made it up!

The point is this: just because you or the coachee made it up on the spur of the moment it does not mean it will not work. Indeed, your unconscious mind may be creating the ideal solution, and if the coachee is willing to take a chance on something new and unknown it might work extremely well. This willingness to make it up and try it out is the essence of co-creation.

LANGUAGE

Language is important in coaching. Another key reason why people hire a personal coach is to gain clarity on a particular issue. Such clarity is gained through the processes of listening, clarifying (above) and by the use of language. The coach and coachee together explore the most appropriate way to define or describe the situation until it is crystal clear what the coachee thinks/feels/needs/wants and/or understands. This can happen in conjunction with clarifying (above). The coachee may be attempting to describe a situation or a feeling. The coach may mirror what the coachee has said then ask: 'What word would describe that feeling you mentioned?'

Together coach and coachee explore different words and phrases until the coachee arrives at an accurate description of their situation. Again this leads to greater clarity which, in turn, leads to effective decision-making.

Drawing a coachee's attention to their use of language is extremely effective in 're-framing' or encouraging a paradigm shift. We may hold a negative world-view or core belief which we have carried since childhood and which we have never challenged. This may be reflected in our negative language and / or negative self-talk. This is evident when we hear colleagues express views such as 'I could never do that', or, even worse, 'I'm too stupid'.

During coaching sessions a coachee will often repeat long-held negative assumptions such as: 'I'm too bossy', 'I'm too fat', 'I'm too tall', 'I'm too short'. Part of challenging these negative core beliefs is to point out the coachee's negative language and to request that they re-frame their view by adopting positive language. It takes time to change long-established patterns, so this would happen over a number of coaching sessions, with the coach pointing out whenever the coachee slips back into their 'old' negative pattern. Sometimes this is used in conjunction with positive affirmations.

The 'wipe-out' game

This is an exercise you can try for yourself. I call it the 'wipe-out' game. As soon as you become aware that you are experiencing a negative thought such as 'I'll never do this', turn it around to its positive opposite. So, 'I'll never do this' becomes 'I WILL do this'. Say this out loud six times. Completely 'wipe-out' your negative thought by replacing each negative thought with six positive affirmations. Do this every time you notice a negative thought.

I once coached a runner who was training for a marathon by running up hills. One day she came to a particularly steep and challenging hill and was saying to herself: 'I want to do this, I'm going to do this', yet it was still a struggle. As soon as she changed what she was saying to a more definite, 'I will do this', she suddenly found it easier to run up that hill.

LISTENING

As coaches we probably spend 80% of our time actively listening. Active listening does not come naturally and requires our full attention. If we are planning what we are going to say next, as in normal conversation, we cannot be fully listening. Active listening demands that we listen fully to the speaker without an agenda of our own and without planning our response. We let the speaker know we are listening fully by nodding or making sounds such as 'uh-uh' or 'mmm' periodically. When the speaker has finished, or after a significant pause, we may repeat back just exactly what we heard them say (a technique known as mirroring) to check that we heard correctly.

LOVE

Love is not a word which appears very often in healthcare texts – and perhaps it should. If we are in healthcare practice the chances are that we do the work we do out of love. What do we mean by this? We certainly do not mean romantic love, the kind where we 'fall in love' and choose a sexual partner. Peck distinguishes between active and passive love. He explains that romantic love is a passive process, something we experience that is beyond our conscious control, and which is linked directly to sexual attraction and propagation of the species. Active love, on the other hand, is something we choose to do. He defines love as:

> *the will to extend one's self for the purpose of nurturing one's own or another's spiritual growth.*
>
> *(Peck, 1990)*

In this sense, the coach must possess willingness, ability, and make a conscious effort to love both themselves and their coachees. In this way they nurture their own, and their coachee's, overall development. During a workshop recently I heard another coach say: 'the only requirement of a coach is self-love'. Once we have this we have something of real value to offer our coachees.

MAKE THE COACHEE RIGHT

Some coaching schools refer to 'making the client (coachee) right' and suggest that a coach should make the coachee feel that they are always right, even if they are wrong (CoachU, 1999). What can this mean? This paradoxical view that they are right even when they are wrong is another way of emphasising unconditional positive regard and the view that people do whatever they feel is right for them in the moment. So, even if someone is about to do something illegal, they are still doing what they feel is 'right' for them, even though it is not legally or even morally considered 'right'.

MEDITATION

I mention meditation here because it is a time-honoured technique for calming the mind and improving concentration. It is extremely useful in developing our presence (below). This is achieved by controlled thinking. A meditation which I often recommend can, despite its simplicity, be quite difficult to achieve for people with active minds. That is the point. Try it for yourself and, afterwards, note in your journal what your experience is. What was meditation like for you? What effect, if any, has it had on your levels of concentration elsewhere in your life?

EXERCISE

Sit in a chair with your back well supported. Close your eyes. Breathe in and out deeply and slowly. With each breath, feel your body relax. Rest your hands gently in your lap. Now imagine a blue triangle with equal sides like a pyramid. Hold it in your attention with your imagination. Allow nothing else to wander into your attention except your blue triangle. We cannot stop our thoughts intruding. Indeed, if you try it seems to happen all the more. Rather, just notice each time your mind wanders and gently bring it back to your blue triangle. Be gentle with yourself. It is your mind's job to think – it's what it does best! If you become tense, frustrated, angry with yourself and/or pressure yourself, you will be less able to concentrate. If your mind wanders, as soon as you notice, gently remind yourself to come back to the triangle.

Try for one minute at first, then increase your time daily. To experience the full benefits of meditation it is best practised on a daily basis.

(I am keen to hear your experience of this exercise. If you are willing, please e-mail your feedback to ruth@dreamcoach.co.uk)

METAPHOR

The use of metaphor, or indeed any technique which offers a mental picture, is invaluable in coaching. As coachees develop and make enormous shifts in their basic viewpoint they will inevitably reach plateaux in their understanding from time to time. A skilled coach creates metaphors which relate to the coachee's personal situation with the aim of illuminating a new concept and shifting the coachee to a new level of awareness. It is also a valuable fieldwork exercise to request the coachee to create their own metaphor.

Metaphors speak to the unconscious, the part of the brain which often holds the answers.

META-VIEW

This is where the coach looks at the overall perspective and places the coachee's current situation in a wider context. Often we are aware of being too 'close' to a situation to see the wider context ourselves. We are too involved and can become narrow in our thinking. We might speak of 'not being able to see the wood for the trees'. The coach is in an ideal position to look at the 'meta-view' – the big picture – and lend a sense of perspective to the coachee's situation.

MODELLING

Modelling, or being a role model, is another invaluable part of the coach's role. Often people will hire a personal coach for this reason – simply because they model personal skills and attributes that a coachee cannot learn elsewhere. Social and interpersonal skills, such as setting personal boundaries, can be modelled within the coaching relationship.

OPINION

We have an opinion and it is not only perfectly acceptable, it is possibly even desirable, to share it provided we have asked permission and the coachee knows that it is just our opinion and not any kind of 'expert' advice. This is related to articulating the truth (above), challenging (above), intuition (above) and 'the edge' (below). Indeed, we have an obligation as coaches, in the name of speaking our truth, to share our opinions. This might be in the context of challenging a coachee on a belief with which we disagree.

For example, I had a coachee with a great fear of death. Not for herself but for her loved ones. At the time, the political climate was such that war was likely and she worried that her sons may be conscripted. Her fear was not of death itself but of the terrible pain and suffering they would (in her opinion) undergo in the last few moments of life. I felt it was my duty to share my opinion that whilst I cannot know for certain that death is painless, from my observations of being with people who have died, the reverse seems true. They appear to be overcome with a peaceful serenity just before death. In sharing this I made it absolutely clear that this was just my opinion, based on my personal experience.

PRESENCE

This is related to 'being with' (above). As coaches, we aim to be always fully present in the moment. In the present moment. This means our attention is not on the past, what we did last night, or five minutes ago, or what we may do in the future. We are fully present in this moment, with our coachee. This takes a special kind of attention and concentration and does not come easily or naturally. When we do achieve it successfully, those around us become aware of our presence. They detect something in our manner. The Oxford English Dictionary refers to presence as 'a person's force of personality' (Pearsall and Trumble, 1996).

Yet in coaching we are not imposing anything on anyone. We are using this same 'force' to create an environment in which our coachees can thrive. It is the quality of our attention, rather than the force of our personality, which creates the presence in coaching.

I recall a story which illustrates this quality perfectly. Two Buddhist monks were raking over some ground in a garden. After some time, one of the monks turned to the other and said:

'Brother, we have been raking for hours now and still my area is covered in stones while in yours the earth is finely raked with no stones left. How can this be?'

The second monk replied:

'You are not fully present. You may be here but your mind is thinking about our meditation later today, what we will have for dinner this evening, how well I am raking my area. Is this not so?'

The first monk answered:

'Yes, that is correct.'

To which the second monk replied:

'When you are fully present, your area will be raked as finely as mine.'

This story beautifully illustrates the important point that when we are fully present in the moment, our attention is fully focused on what we are doing, and excellence is the natural result. It is no accident that the characters in the above illustration are monks. True presence is difficult to achieve unless we are skilled in some kind of technique for managing our naturally wandering thoughts.

Our attention span is presumed to be anywhere from 10 to 20 minutes. Under normal circumstances this makes 'being fully present' impossible for a 55 minute coaching session. To most new coaches I recommend meditation (above), or indeed any technique which expands our ability to concentrate, as a method of practising being fully present for increasingly longer periods of time. When we are present we have presence.

QUESTIONING

Questioning is considered an essential aspect of the art of coaching. It is sometimes referred to as effective questioning, artful questioning or powerful questioning. In their enthusiasm to have a profound effect on their coachees this is where many coaches feel their influence lies. Undoubtedly a well-placed question might result in a huge shift in perspective on the part of the coachee, and this is often despite the coach's intention rather than because of it.

It is almost impossible to have a profound effect on somebody simply by trying to. Think back to some of the people who have had a profound effect on you in your lifetime. Were they trying to have this effect?

I prefer to caution against trying too hard in this respect. As we gain experience in coaching our questions come naturally, out of our curiosity and our genuine desire to facilitate our coachee's development. Trying too hard often results in ineffective coaching since the coachee may feel they are subject to interrogation. I hear horror stories of novice coaches 'pinning' people into a corner at parties, coaching them without permission and, as if that wasn't bad enough, interrogating them. This is not coaching!

To some coaches the 'great coaching question' becomes the elusive 'holy grail' of coaching, and I admit I fell into this category when I first set up my coaching practice. I believed that if I could only find that one profound question, all my coachee's problems would just melt away and the solutions would neatly fall into place.

While my attention was on thinking up this question I was not fully listening and neither was I fully present. In my various attempts to generate the 'great coaching question' my coachees must have also felt they were interrogated at times. In reality we are often only aware that we have asked a great question after we have asked it.

We know we have asked a great coaching question when:

- it feels spontaneous
- it is inspired by listening to the coachee
- it comes from a genuine love of, and concern for, the coachee
- the client has to think before answering
- the client is silent
- we are naturally curious
- the client shifts (a paradigm / perspective shift or they move to another level in their development)
- the client is enthused, inspired and / or creates solutions where before they were stuck.

REFRAMING

Reframing is where we place another perspective on an issue, concept or word. An example was mentioned briefly in Chapter 2 in relation to negative core beliefs. When we reframe something we describe real qualities and point out attributes that the coachee may not have seen herself, so that she sees it from a different perspective.

Perhaps someone has always been told they are 'too bossy', and believes this to be a negative quality. A coach might say: 'Let's reframe this. In what circumstances would being bossy be a desirable, if not essential, quality?'

In common language, reframing might also be thought of as putting a positive 'spin' on the issue, though this is an unnecessarily superficial view of an extremely useful technique. In requesting the coachee to reframe a long-held core belief we enable them to see a wider perspective and accept that their belief is based on an assumption which may have been made in childhood and which can no longer be held to be 'truth' or reality from an adult perspective.

REQUESTING

Requesting is an essential skill in the art of effective coaching. This is what keeps the coachee moving towards their objective. The language is quite specific. We begin our requests quite literally with the words: 'I request that you...'

This is effective in gaining the coachee's commitment to change and moving them forward. A suggestion does not carry the same emphasis as a strong request.

EXERCISE

Compare these two sentences:

- 'I suggest you visit your doctor sometime for a health check.'
- 'I request you visit your doctor for a health check. Are you willing to do that?'

What do you notice between the two sentences?

The second sentence makes a request, then asks a question which demands a reply: 'Are you willing to do that?'

The request is not a demand. A coachee always has choices. She can agree to the request, decline, or offer a modified response such as: 'No, I won't see the doctor, but I'm willing to go and speak with the nurse practitioner.' She has committed to action rather than just leaving it open which, over time, may mean she simply never gets around to it.

If you were the coach in the above example, how would you respond if the coachee simply replies with 'No'?

Write down some of your possible responses.

(I am keen to hear your experience of this exercise. If you are willing, please e-mail your feedback to ruth@dreamcoach.co.uk)

The goal is to have the coachee commit to some action on their own behalf so an appropriate response would be something like: 'What are you willing to do, then?'

It is perfectly acceptable for a coachee to refuse the coach's request. However, for the coaching to be effective, the coachee needs to take some action, so the coach always aims for a commitment to action of some kind. The coach might ask: 'What are you going to commit to this week to move you forward on this?'

In making a request, the coach is aiming for a commitment to action. The request then needs to be followed up with questions that cement the commitment and place it within the context of a timeframe: 'Are you willing to do that?', followed by: 'Great, when will you do it?'

Requesting is unambiguous and unequivocal. The request is powerful and commands our coachee's attention. The request gives our coachees an opportunity to move forward on an issue by taking action, yet it affords them the opportunity to avoid making the decision about which action to take. This can be useful in overcoming long-held resistance or fear if they are ready and willing to take the chance. Instead of asking: 'What do you want to do to move forward on this?' the coach goes one step further and states: 'I request that you do this.' Again, obtaining permission is recommended. In a long-term established coaching relationship, permission may be implied, but it is still wise to ask: 'May I make a request of you?'

SILENCE

Silence is rarely empty. We 'fill' silence with our thoughts, images, vision, inspiration, intuition and feelings. Developing our awareness of these depends on our learning to be comfortable with silence and sit with it. As coaches we learn to respect and be comfortable with silence. Silence can be a gift. When our coachee is silent they may be thinking. They may be feeling. They may be reflecting. They are experiencing themselves. When our coachee is silent, often the best way to coach them is to be fully present and wait. Let the coachee be the first to break the silence. Silence in coaching is golden. It is a golden space into which come valuable insights, inspirations and intuitions. Learn to respect silence and the gifts it can bring.

SHIFT

Shift is another term commonly quoted in a coaching context. Coaching texts often refer to coachees 'shifting' and making a huge 'shift' (CoachU, 1999). In this context it refers to a stage of development. This can be a major insight, a shift in perspective, a paradigm shift and/or a noticeable move to another level of learning. For example, in terms of learning a skill, we may 'shift' from novice to skilled, from skilled to expert, and then from expert to mastery of any given subject.

STRUCTURE

This has been covered in Chapter 2 so I will simply recap a couple of points here. In a coaching context, structure refers to the practical steps that are put into place to ensure objectives are met. It is the framework within which the required objective(s) will take place. This might be physical structure, like organising our personal accounts into a filing system, or it may be a series of daily action steps which we will take to ensure our objectives are met. It is the responsibility of the coach and coachee together to co-create this structure.

THE EDGE

This is an unusual term which is often used in coaching and possibly derives from a business or corporate context. The edge is defined as:

Truth spoken directly and with compassion

(CoachU, 1999)

Sometimes coaches are described as 'having an edge', meaning they are forthright and direct. It is always worth remembering that the word compassion is included in this definition. The edge is commonly used when confronting or challenging a client and can be threatening unless exercised with great skill and compassion.

VALUES BASING

This is another unusual term which you may come across in coaching texts, especially if they originate in the USA. It refers to basing the coaching around the coachee's core values. In the UK we might refer to this as a value-centred style.

Core values are those things which we value most in life. It is possible to live and work out of alignment with our values, and many of us do, but when we do so we experience a sense that something is missing or that we are not being 'true to ourselves'. If the coachee is considering a major career change, it is certainly worth encouraging them to identify their core values, and whether the change will bring them more into alignment with their values. Sooner or later most coachees will undertake a review of their values. Having a strong sense of our values, and the ability to integrate them into our daily lives, is essential to our sense of fulfilment.

VISION

Coaches are naturally interested in developing their coachee's vision. This might be a vision for their business or career, such as where they see themselves in two years' time, or it may be a vision for their ideal life. The vision is our coachee's ultimate destination. It is where they are heading. Their vision is what will pull them forward. Experienced coaches focus on the coachee's vision at the beginning of a coaching relationship and refer back to it frequently throughout the coaching period. A vision should be capable of evolving with the coachee and as such continue to pull them forward. Powerful visions attract like a magnet.

VISUAL DISPLAYS

The axiom 'a picture paints a thousand words' is so apt. Visual images are extremely powerful and are retained in our memories much more readily than words and language. The advertising industry understands this. Consider how powerful a visual image can be on a poster campaign or a television commercial.

EXERCISE

Take a moment to recall powerful images you have seen today. What made them so powerful? Did they provoke an emotional response in you?

(I am keen to hear your experience of this exercise. If you are willing, please e-mail your feedback to ruth@dreamcoach.co.uk)

As mentioned earlier, coaches will try to invoke a visual image if possible through the use of metaphor to illustrate a powerful point or to help the coachee to shift. Visual imagery can also be used as a reminder of our goals to keep us on track.

It may be helpful to encourage a coachee to work with a visioning board. A visioning board is a notice board, or cork board, placed in a prominent position where the coachee will see it every day. Upon this board the coachee pins lots of visual images which relate to their vision. They may even write out their vision in large letters and pin this in the centre of the board. These images can come from any source: magazines, newspapers, family photos and / or websites. The coachee effectively builds a 'collage' with them. This becomes a daily visual reminder of where they are headed: their vision.

VISUALISATION

Visualisation is another powerful imaging technique which uses the power of the coachee's own imagination to enable them to step into their own future. In a visualisation they are encouraged to create as real a scenario as their imagination will allow by including as many senses as they can muster: seeing, hearing, feeling, touching, smelling and tasting. Visualisation enables them to 'live' the experience as vividly as possible and connect with their 'future' self.

This technique connects people, in a vivid and realistic way, with their own potential. This is also what we do when we are daydreaming. Often we will daydream that we are in a role or position that we desire, but when we 'awake' or return from our daydream we allow our negative beliefs to convince us it is only a 'pipedream' that we could not achieve in reality. The reality is that daydreaming and visualisation are powerful learning tools. In a visualisation or daydream we get to rehearse the necessary skills that we would need in the real situation. We tap into the power of play, like children do when they 'play' at being a popstar, for example. This powerful technique enables us to identify the required knowledge and skills, and then practice them. It moves us toward a greater degree of competency in any area.

EXERCISE

Visualise a position or scenario that you desire and really allow your daydream to take over. Let your imagination run wild!

How do you feel? What are you doing? How are you behaving?

(I am keen to hear your experience of this exercise. If you are willing, please e-mail your feedback to ruth@dreamcoach.co.uk)

Visualisation is especially effective with interpersonal skills, which is why rehearsals work so well for acting and public speaking.

WALK-THROUGH

Once the coachee has identified a goal and/or vision, the coach walks through it with them to develop the vision further. Together they will explore this alternative reality and how closely it matches the coachee's core values. Once a vision becomes this real, coachees often experience resistance and it is important to look at this and discover what might be holding them back from fulfilling their vision.

The International Coach Federation (ICF) is a professional organisation for coaches based in the USA. Though it is not an officially recognised regulatory body it offers some preliminary standards and guidelines for the coaching profession. It strives for greater quality in coaching by setting standards for coach training. With this aim in mind the ICF has identified 11 core coaching competencies (Figure 3.1) which it groups together under the following four headings:

Setting the foundation

Co-creating the relationship

Communicating effectively, and

Facilitating learning and results.

(International Coach Federation, 2002)

This helps to place the wide range of coaching skills and competencies into some kind of context. Though there are many coach training schools throughout the UK, there is no officially recognised regulatory body at the time of writing, though this may change.

Coaching Core Competencies

The following eleven core coaching competencies were developed to support greater understanding about the skills and approaches used within today's coaching profession as defined by the ICF. They will also support you in calibrating the level of alignment between the coach-specific training expected and the training you have experienced.

Finally, these competencies were used as the foundation for the ICF Credentialing process examination. The core competencies are grouped into four clusters according to those that fit together logically based on common ways of looking at the competencies in each group. The groupings and individual competencies are not weighted – they do not represent any kind of priority in that they are all core or critical for any competent coach to demonstrate.

A. SETTING THE FOUNDATION

1. Meeting ethical guidelines and professional standards
2. Establishing the coaching agreement

B. CO-CREATING THE RELATIONSHIP

3. Establishing trust and intimacy with the client
4. Coaching presence

C. COMMUNICATING EFFECTIVELY

5. Active listening
6. Powerful questioning
7. Direct communication

D. FACILITATING LEARNING AND RESULTS

8. Creating awareness
9. Designing actions
10. Planning and goal setting
11. Managing progress and accountability

(ICF Internet document located at
http://www.coachfederation.org/credentialing/en/core.htm)

Figure 3.1 ICF core coaching competencies (Reproduced, with permission, from the International Coach Federation, 2002)

4

You as coachee: the coaching experience

Each of us must be the change we want to see in the world.

Mahatma Gandhi

This chapter focuses on us as coachees. It highlights the changes that we could make when we choose to experience coaching as a tool for our own personal development.

So far we have discussed the role of coaching in implementing change. Paradoxically, rather than inherently changing us, coaching helps us to define with greater clarity who we are and who we are not. In this sense, coaching in itself does not change us as much as introduce us to our real selves. Coaching offers a nurturing environment in which we may choose to make changes in our lives as we develop this greater sense of self and re-orientate our lives to come into alignment with our 'true' self. The coaching process draws our attention to who we are being when we act out roles that we have adopted throughout our lives. Through self-observation and self-inquiry we challenge these roles and identify which ones no longer fit with our sense of who we are. In some roles, we may have lost our sense of self. This is a common phenomenon in healthcare professionals – we become so inextricably linked with our role that we lose sight of who we are. Many healthcare professionals have commented that they 'don't know who they are' anymore. They have become synonymous with their role as a healthcare professional and have lost their sense of a separate self outside of the role. They feel they have become the role in that they have become defined by what they do rather than who they are. This is reflected in language such as: 'I am a midwife.'

If we allow ourselves to be defined by what we do, but then, for whatever reason, we are no longer able to do it, what happens to who we are? Who or what do we become? More importantly, what happens to our self-esteem, our sense of worth and our intrinsic value?

In terms of managing our own career, there may be nothing more essential than recognising our deepest feelings about what we do – and what changes might make us more truly satisfied with our work.

(Goleman, 1996)

When we choose to hire a personal coach, we are investing in ourselves. Choosing our coach is part of the process. This differs tremendously from being coached professionally, either by our peers (peer coaching), our manager and/or a designated coach or mentor, in a number of respects. When we experience coaching with a personal coach we notice straight away that we are working with someone who has no attachment to the organisational or professional objectives. We may even switch jobs or careers and continue working with the same coach. We can establish a long-term trusting relationship, and co-create a nurturing environment in which we can grow.

The process of coaching, which includes self-management, self-inquiry, self-discovery, self-observation and increasing self-awareness, gradually brings us toward the level of self-actualisation described by Maslow (Figure 2.1). We become clearer about our own values, unique gifts and talents, indeed the very things that make us who we are. We develop clarity between who we are and what we do. Rather than changing who we are, coaching enables us to become aware of the illusion that we are the roles we play, and allows who we really are to surface. We develop a sense of self, and a realisation of our intrinsic self-worth that is not dependent on any outside person or role for validation. We set strong personal boundaries for ourselves once we recognise that this 'self' we have discovered is valuable to us and worth protecting. Our self-esteem increases. Our confidence increases. We become more focused and less drained by distractions in our lives. We have fewer distractions because we value our time, have strong boundaries in place, and have structures in place to manage our time effectively. We achieve more, feel less tired, and have more time to spend on ourselves too.

We can see that wherever we are on Maslow's hierarchy of need (Figure 2.1) would influence the coaching focus, which is why it is important for coaching to always be client-led. If our needs are physiological and safety-related, the coaching focus would be on our learning self-management and putting structures in place to fulfil and maintain those needs. If our needs are social-orientated, the coaching focus may be on developing our interpersonal skills, networking and raising emotional literacy. As we move towards esteem needs, we may find the coaching focus is on becoming our selves, developing a strong sense of self and learning to acknowledge and value our selves. When our needs tend towards self-actualisation, we may find the coaching focus centres around our core values and integrating these into our lives for a sense of fulfilment. Provided the coaching session is always coachee-led, and the coach is detached from the outcome, the coaching focus will be appropriate for the coachee's current needs.

RESISTANCE

When we make any kind of change, large or small, desired or unwelcome, we experience a degree of anxiety. Think about it for a moment. Even when we go on that long-awaited and much-desired holiday of a lifetime. We experience anxiety. Do we need vaccinations? Will the tickets arrive on time? Is our passport up to date? Do we need a visa? Have we remembered everything, or is there some glaringly obvious oversight? This much anxiety is generated from something as potentially pleasurable as a holiday which we have probably looked forward to for months, if not years. The anxiety is caused by our moving from the familiar to the unfamiliar. When our minds become over-active, running through a check-list of things to remember, we are attempting to grasp control of the situation. Imagine how much anxiety we experience when faced with a change that has been initiated externally, by someone else, a change that is not our desired choice, is beyond our control and will almost certainly have repercussions for us. High level anxiety. We may not recognise it as such. We may use the term 'stress'. Whichever term we use, on an emotional level, it is a greater or lesser degree of anxiety that we are experiencing. We lose conscious control and our 'emotional brain' is in charge again (see EQ Chapter 2).

The phrase 'resistance to change' has become almost a cliché in management circles. In some organisations it is perceived to signal a lack of commitment to organisational objectives. This view is unhelpful and denotes an ignorance of the normal human response to change of any kind. We are ALL resistant to change. Resistance arises from within us, and is a perfectly normal response to change. Even when we are forging ahead with changes that are self-initiated and desirable, as in our holiday example (above) or a promotion, we experience resistance. We get 'cold feet'. We begin to doubt ourselves. We experience anxiety and fear which becomes evident in our worrying thoughts:

Why did I book this holiday?

What have I let myself in for?

I hate flying – maybe I should cancel and stay at home where I feel safe.

Why did I apply for this job? I'm not sure I'm up to it.

When we cancel, have 'second thoughts', and change our minds it is because our anxiety has reached such a level as to become uncomfortable. It becomes apparent to us that the fastest and most logical way to ease our discomfort is to remove the source, even if that means cancelling our holiday. A decision which might seem illogical to an outside observer makes perfect sense to us because we directly experience our discomfort, feelings and emotions, and so we understand the decision to relieve the discomfort.

In a workplace situation we may experience a gradual increase in our anxiety, as minor changes are introduced one at a time, or we may experience a sudden surge of anxiety as huge sweeping changes are proposed. When anxiety becomes unbearable many people will simply leave.

Resistance to change is our protective response to a feeling of fear and anxiety. It is part of our natural defence mechanism which protects us against stress and ill-health. Resistance tells us when we are changing too fast, too often, or are reaching beyond our capabilities, and have not taken enough time to assimilate existing changes. When it is viewed this way, we can see how resistance protects us against stress or the change fatigue brought about by continual change in the workplace. Resistance is a warning signal to us to slow down, and to take time to acclimatise to one set of changes before embarking upon another.

Acknowledging resistance and anxiety is part of the coaching process. It enables us, as coachees, to recognise where we feel resistance within ourselves and how to interpret the signs. When resistance shows up it is a signal that we need to look at how we are proposing to change. Are we moving too fast? Do we need to slow things down to give ourselves time to assimilate? Do we need support?

As coachees, we experience resistance many times as we confront our fears, challenge our selves, push back our frontiers and do bigger and better things than we ever would have dreamed possible. Coaches become very familiar with resistance in coachees and recognise it as a good sign for two reasons. First, the coachee who is experiencing resistance has probably already stepped out of her 'comfort zone' and made huge changes. This is worth acknowledging. Secondly it is a wonderful gauge to let the coach know not to push the coachee too hard, or to caution the coachee not to push herself too hard. Reaching for goals which are beyond our current level of skill and expertise can be a form of self-sabotage. Rather than learning through gradual steps it is known to coaches that some people will over-stretch themselves and, when they fail, use this as reinforcement of their belief that they will be unable to achieve their goal.

Resistance becomes a useful yardstick to allow us to stay in the 'flow state' (see Chapter 2) of peak performance. When we are resistant, we know it is time to step back and become comfortable with our new level of skill before we attempt to forge ahead with more change.

WHO DO WE BECOME UNDER STRESS?

Most of us, especially in the healthcare professions, like to think that we are calm and in control under stress and that it does not affect our performance. However, our ability to keep a cool head under stress and get the job done does not mean we are unaffected. Our ability to maintain a reassuring, cool, calm exterior only disguises the anxiety that we feel. It may be the case that we are suppressing our emotions and this does not render us immune to the physical effects of stress. We may have a calm exterior and rising blood pressure. In stressful working environments, anxiety runs high, though it may not be visible. The higher our anxiety, the more our performance *is* affected. Our ability to think clearly deteriorates in direct relation to rising anxiety levels (Goleman, 1996).

As mentioned earlier, we have predictable patterns of behaviour that we adopt under stress. Often they are patterns that we established at an early age and, as such, they do not reflect an intelligent, mature outlook. They are largely driven by our 'emotional brain', which means our conscious, thinking, rational, cortex has been by-passed and we are in an adapted version of our own personal 'fear/fight/flight' response. We are in an emotionally-charged state and, because of our limited capacity to think clearly, we resort to fixed behaviour patterns which have become familiar to us (also see 'polarised relationships', Chapter 2).

In our childhood and youth we learn effective ways to overcome our emotional distress, anxiety and discomfort. We learn behaviour patterns which then become our first line of defence when under stress. So if, for example, we learned to 'take over' and overfunction, 'fixing' everyone else's problems for them and dispensing advice, this may be a fixed pattern within us that we resort to when stressed. The more stressed we are, the more exaggerated this aspect of our behaviour becomes. If we are normally viewed by our colleagues as assertive and good at organising, we may be seen as intolerably bossy when under stress. A pattern which may have been very effective when we developed it at age 13 may be completely inappropriate in our adult working relationships at the age of 43.

The usual suspects

At this point I would like to introduce you to a cast of characters who may sound familiar to you: The Superhero, The Judge, The Tyrant, The 'Lone Ranger', The People Pleaser and The Martyr.

There is also a full supporting cast, but for our purposes here let us examine some of the main characters that may show up when we are under stress. We met 'The Superhero' briefly above. The Superhero is the archetypal overfunctioner. The 'fixer'. This is the part of ourselves that wants to be a hero. When we are in Superhero mode we want to save the world and everyone in it. If we have a Superhero aspect it is most likely to step in when things get rough and 'take over' to solve everyone else's problems. It is the Superhero who is often thought of as wonderfully assertive and organised by some, and intolerably bossy, overbearing and unbearable by others. On first reading this, you may be thinking about all the people you know who fit into this category. As tempting as it may be to diagnose your family, friends, colleagues, supervisors, manager and/or peers, I encourage you to recognise which aspects you can identify within yourself. As you read the next section, I invite you to become the calm, observer of self that we mentioned earlier.

The Judge

The Judge lives within us all. It is otherwise known as our inner critic, our Gremlin (Carson, 1990), internal saboteur, and many other names. This is the voice inside our head that bombards us with negative self-talk:

Why did I ever think I could do this?

Who do I think I am?

I can't do this.

I shouldn't have done it that way.

Maybe I was wrong.

The stronger our inner Judge's voice, the lower our self-esteem will be.

The Judge does not want us to try anything new. The Judge is quite happy sticking to what is familiar, and being an advocate for every 'should', 'ought' and 'must' we ever heard.

Shoulds, oughts and musts always have their origins externally. We may have internalised them over time, but whenever we hear ourselves thinking 'I should do this' the origin is usually someone else and not ourselves. They are red flag words to a coach because they signal where we are not being true to our selves and may be acting out of habit, duty or obligation. It is not necessarily wrong to act out of duty or obligation. This might mean we are acting responsibly. When we hear ourselves thinking those words it is always worth challenging our thinking, to see whether we are being driven by an outdated behaviour pattern that is a remnant of our past and which no longer serves us. The Judge is the internalised voice of our parents, siblings, peers – indeed every critic we have ever heard, all rolled into one.

The Tyrant

A close relative of the Judge, 'should', 'ought' and 'must' are also familiar words in the Tyrant's vocabulary. If you have an inner Tyrant, you will be familiar with phrases such as:

I should clean up more.

I should exercise.

I should do my degree.

I should be a better mother.

I should earn more.

I'm lazy.

The Tyrant is never satisfied, and drives us forward mercilessly. If you feel guilty when resting and feel as if you are 'doing nothing', you may well have an inner Tyrant. If you have an inner Tyrant, you may well be a workaholic driving yourself relentlessly towards burnout.

The Lone Ranger

You will easily recognise if you have a 'Lone Ranger' aspect if you find it difficult to ask for and accept help from others. If you refuse too quickly, automatically, out of habit, when others offer help, you have a tendency to be a Lone Ranger. It is the Lone Ranger within us that will struggle on alone when others could help, and still we just cannot bring ourselves to ask for the help we need.

The Lone Ranger may find herself using language such as:

It's OK, I can manage.

You can't rely on other people.

If you want a job doing well, you have to do it yourself.

The Lone Ranger is usually very capable, since she would rather learn how to do everything herself than ask for help. This aspect of ourselves may also contribute to burnout, especially if combined with a Superhero aspect. In that case, we may be someone who does everything for ourselves and others, yet cannot accept help for ourselves.

The People Pleaser

The People Pleaser needs to be loved, acknowledged, accepted, liked and approved of. The People Pleaser needs to know what others want and need before making a decision, since the motive is to please them. Without this information about others, the People Pleaser is almost paralysed. The People Pleaser is unaccustomed to taking only their own needs into account before making a decision. It is the People Pleaser aspect of ourselves that leads us to over-explain and over-justify our actions. When we do this, we are really saying to the other person: 'Please understand me.' When we care too much what others will think or what their reaction will be, this is the People Pleaser within us.

The Martyr

'Woe is me!' and 'Poor me!' are the call signs of the Martyr. If we are driven by suffering, if we are in love with our own struggle and find ourselves thinking we have it tougher than everyone else, then we have a Martyr living within us. Our inner Martyr is driven by a need for sympathy. Our Martyr not only needs others to know how much we are suffering, but needs them to know that we are suffering the most: 'You think you've got it bad? Wait until you hear what happened to me.'

We may, if we are courageous enough to look closely, find that we have elements of each of these characters. We all recognise The Judge. We can identify with self-criticism. In recognising these 'archetypes' we begin to note that they are not 'us', but rather aspects of ourselves which may become exaggerated when we are under pressure. We could include Victim and Bully here too. It takes courage to willingly look at ourselves and acknowledge: 'I am that.'

Observation, self-awareness and self-acceptance are important stages in our journey to self-actualisation and emotional literacy. In the coaching process, this is at the level of checking our current reality. Until we know this about ourselves, we will be unable to change. We need this information about ourselves before we can make a decision about how to be different.

For example, if I do not want to be a victim any longer, what information do I need in order to change? I need to understand in what context, under what circumstances, I become a victim. What happens to me? How does my behaviour change, and where do I give up my power? I obtain this information by simply observing myself in different situations. I need to recognise the choices I make, or do not make, that lead me to fall into victimhood. Once I have this information, I can see where I could make different choices. I can begin to choose how I would like to behave instead.

If we become judgemental of ourselves in this process we are likely to shrink away from it, and slow down or halt our progress. We are much more likely to persevere in this arduous task by working with a supportive coach in a positive, nurturing environment. This helps us to acknowledge our courage and to feel proud of ourselves throughout this process.

Working with a coach to develop a greater sense of 'self' may seem at first to be an abstract concept which is unrelated to our work. Yet the process of 'de-selfing' (Lerner, 1989) or, put another way, the problem of not fully maturing into our self, leads us to experience problems in all our relationships, including those at work. Within polarised relationships (see Chapter 2), where one person overfunctions and another may underfunction, the underfunctioning person is 'de-selfing', in that they become less of their true selves. When we 'de-self' within a relationship we become less of who we are and the other person develops a sense of 'pseudo-self', or a false sense of self, at our expense. De-selfing is part of the process of underfunctioning. It is an aspect of underfunctioning behaviour in which we become 'less' of ourselves and (albeit unconsciously) invite the other person to overfunction on our behalf.

The following example illustrates how de-selfing affects who we become in a relationship. Julie called me for some coaching because, in her words, she was being 'bullied at work' and she wanted to explore what she could do to change. Julie is a Registered Nurse working in a private nursing home. She is well educated, with a first degree, and is currently working toward a

Masters degree. Julie believes her manager to be less well educated, possibly to GCSE level, and she feels this is the source of some jealousy. This particular manager criticises Julie's work and double-checks her decisions, which leaves Julie feeling undermined.

Julie says she never mentions her education or personal development needs at work, and often remains quiet. This affects her work, since she takes a passive role and prefers to keep professional opinions, innovations and ideas about potential practice improvements to herself, for fear of ridicule and/or criticism. She is very conscious of how she speaks and presents herself in the presence of her manager. She says:

I know I play down my achievements – I don't want to wind her up and have her think I'm boasting.

Julie is beginning to take a de-selfing position in this relationship. In this context, she is being less of herself by effectively 'hiding' aspects of her self. She modifies her behaviour in a misguided attempt to improve the relationship. Her reaction is based on a couple of assumptions. First, she makes the common assumption that she knows why her manager behaves this way. She attributes a motive to the behaviour that she observes in the manager (also see attribution theory, Chapter 2). Secondly, she has expectations of her manager. Based on her first assumption, she also assumes that if she can avoid mentioning her education, and indeed pretend she is less intelligent, then she can lead her manager to improve her behaviour toward her. This never works. It is the beginning of a polarised relationship where the other person gains 'pseudo-self' (a false sense of self) at the expense of the de-selfed person. One person in the relationship overfunctions and the other begins to underfunction. This could be a pattern that Julie developed in childhood and one to which she resorts when under stress because it is familiar to her. In polarised relationships, our thinking also becomes narrow. We think 'either/or'. This is typified in the axiom: 'If you can't beat 'em, join 'em.'

Julie may not be aware that other options exist. Another person in exactly the same circumstances may not have reacted to the manager's behaviour by de-selfing. If prolonged over time, Julie could find herself in an entrenched underfunctioning position.

Note that, in this example, Julie's attention has largely been on her manager. She has effectively observed, judged and diagnosed her manager's 'problem', and prescribed a 'solution'. The coaching process, through inquiry, encourages Julie to become an observer of herself. To observe her own behaviour until she is aware of, and familiar with, the pattern in this relationship – and indeed, all her relationships. Through avid self-observation Julie will come to recognise who she is being in each of the relationships in her life. She may notice that this relationship with her manager parallels another relationship in her life. The coaching process will enable her to recognise where she has choices and could do things differently. Then, the continued support that is present within an ongoing coaching relationship will enable her to have the courage to implement some desired changes.

In a situation that feels hopeless, the coaching process empowers us by helping us to realise where we have choices that can make a difference. Coaching can help us to stop repeating behaviour patterns that are ineffective, and to learn and implement new patterns that are effective.

We all do better when we can de-intensify our anxious focus on the others' problem and put our primary energy into clarifying our own beliefs, convictions, values and priorities, while formulating plans and life goals that are congruent with these.

(Lerner, 1989)

Dr Murray Bowen (1978) identified this reciprocal pattern in relationships and suggested that such behaviour patterns are symptomatic of underground anxiety in a family system. This is known as the Bowen family-systems theory. Lerner (1989) describes how underground anxiety from one relationship, even one that does not directly involve us, can carry over into another. So it is possible, for example, to be carrying underground anxiety about an uncle's death even though we do not feel emotionally close to him and we are quite distant emotionally and geographically. By identifying the source of our anxiety and dealing with that, we reduce the anxiety and problem behaviour within the family system. Underground anxiety is carried throughout entire family systems and is often carried over into relationships outside the family, including those with work colleagues. We may unknowingly be acting out a role within a working relationship with a colleague that is not only based on a behaviour pattern we learned within our own family, but fuelled by continued anxiety within our family. The reverse is also true. We can carry undergound anxiety from our working relationship system into our family. If we need not be directly involved to experience anxiety, then we can see how anxiety about workplace bullying (or indeed any tension at work), even though it does not involve us directly, can have repercussions throughout all our relationships.

When we occasionally behave out of character, in a professional context, it may be because we are unconsciously anxious about a seemingly unrelated event elsewhere in our family system. This is a normal response to stress and anxiety which we all experience and which is beyond our conscious control. We are no more immune to our emotional responses to stress than we are to any other hormonal response.

Since we cannot change others, the challenge is to improve our relationships and raise our EQ by changing ourselves. The paradox is that in changing ourselves we influence others. We can change our behaviour in a situation and this may lead others to reflect upon and change their behaviour. This is where Lerner (1989) uses the metaphor of dance. If you change your steps, the other person cannot continue doing the same dance. Therefore they probably will change in some way, thought we cannot assume that they will change in a predictable way. We cannot expect that A will lead to B. We may well be a role model and inspire similar changes in them – or we may not. Changing others should not be the motive behind our own change. We must keep our attention on ourselves rather than the other person, and not have expectations of them. If the other person does change their behaviour, it may not be in a way that we approve of, and we must also prepare ourselves for that.

'CHANGE BACK' REACTIONS AND COUNTERMOVES

This is difficult and challenging work, as anything worthwhile usually is. There are consequences to our actions and the other people involved in our relationships may well come up with countermoves of their own. Significant relationships, at home and at work, cannot be changed by a single 'hit and run' manoeuvre. We may initiate changes one day, then feel like we are back where we started the next. We may slide back and forth between our new desired behaviour and our old familiar patterns. We may do this many times before we begin to notice lasting changes in our relationships. As a result, we may appear inconsistent, but we should not allow this to deter us. It is important to keep trying and to be gentle with ourselves as we undergo this process of change.

The other people involved in our relationships will test our resolve to see if we really have changed, and whether these changes are permanent. They will react to our proposed changes. Lerner (1990) describes this as a 'change back' reaction, and at its source is their anxiety. When we make changes in a relationship we cause a degree of anxiety in the other person. If they become angry, silent, or react in some other way, it is because they are experiencing anxiety at the change and what the implications might be for them.

We also experience 'change back' reactions from within ourselves, in the form of resistance. At first we will not be comfortable with the change and may crave the familiar old pattern, even if it is unhealthy for us.

Coaching can be a source of support, motivation and encouragement during this difficult time. We gain a sense of direction by returning to the calm objectivity within the coaching relationship. This enables us to see our role in our relationships with clarity. The coach holds our map and shines the torch for us, but it is up to us to navigate our own path. When coaching is effective, the coach is serving as a mirror and a safe haven where we can both experiment with being ourselves and co-create a plan. Our coach helps us back on track when we feel that our attempts to change entrenched patterns in our relationships have been de-railed. Our coach reminds us that we have embarked upon an enormous task, and that our best chance of progress is to take one step at a time. Our coach helps us to determine which goals are achievable now, and which ones might be more than we are ready for yet. Our coach reminds us to be gentle on ourselves in the process, not to judge ourselves negatively and to give ourselves the space we need to grow. We become less likely to sabotage ourselves by initially taking on too much, then becoming overwhelmed and giving up. This would reinforce any negative belief we have. This is why it is important to keep our goals realistic and achievable. An experienced coach recognises self-sabotage patterns, helps us to recognise how we sabotage ourselves and gently steers us away, showing us an alternative and feasible way forward.

There is no quick fix. Coachees work for months on changing entrenched behaviour patterns. Though simple in theory, these patterns are often very difficult to change in practice, requiring a great deal of motivation, persistence and courage from us. Changes this permanent and effective are never easy or comfortable. Sometimes we feel driven to take challenging steps toward change because we know that not changing would be more difficult and challenging. This drive stems from our innate need to grow. If we do not change, we fear losing our sense of self.

HOW DO WE DISTINGUISH EFFECTIVE ACTION ON OUR PART FROM INEFFECTIVE ACTION?

Often we make attempts to change, or think we do, only to find we have achieved nothing, or seemingly made matters worse. We may give up at this point and return to the previous status quo. This in itself is a common behaviour pattern: repeated ineffective attempts to change which reinforce our belief that we are powerless keep us 'stuck' in the same behaviour patterns. This could be happening for several reasons. We may be sabotaging our own plans (albeit unconsciously). This may be because preserving the status quo benefits us in some way that we may not consciously acknowledge. It takes courage to accept that we might be gaining in some way. For example, if we are a victim, in an underfunctioning role, this can serve us by enabling us to avoid taking responsibility in our lives and making our own decisions. If we allow someone else to make decisions for us, we have someone to blame when life does not go the way we would like it to.

Our goal will be to have relationships with both men and women that do not operate at the expense of the self, and to have a self that does not operate at the expense of the other.

(Lerner, 1989)

Acknowledging our stories

Coaching offers us a place where it is safe to share our own stories with our coach and to acknowledge our journey through life. This enables us to see patterns and an overall trend in our growth. We develop a sense of direction: a sense of where we have come from and what we are heading towards. In developing a stronger sense of self we acknowledge how far we have come and how far we have yet to go. We become aware of and acknowledge our unique strengths and our courage. As we recognise our own values and begin to align our actions with our beliefs, we feel more in integrity. We become more authentic in the process. Others become aware that we are in alignment: we 'practice what we preach'.

When we live in integrity, we become excellent role models for our family, friends, clients, coachees and colleagues. Being authentic lends us an even stronger presence. We are living our own advice, 'taking our own medicine', healing ourselves from within and raising our EQ. We are walking, talking role models with authentic stories to share, based on our own experience and wisdom rather than something we read somewhere. Our coachees sense that we, too, have 'been there' and understand what they are experiencing. This bridges the 'them and us' gap within the practitioner-client relationship. We become partners in healing.

As we develop our authenticity in this way, we shift our awareness and our perspective. We begin to acknowledge that every experience is an opportunity for growth and learning.

When I left the NHS in 1997 I had had enough. I felt exploited, unappreciated, undervalued, overworked, overloaded, burned out, used up and stressed out. All the usual clichés. I felt like I had been wrung out, washed out and hung out to dry. I felt I had nothing left to give. Sound familiar?

How could 'they' do this? How could 'they' take healthy, intelligent people and suck the life out of them? What was going on? The problem seemed clear to me: intimidation and blame were inherent parts of the culture of healthcare in this country. Intimidate people to get the job done, and blame them if things do not go according to plan.

I could not see that I had become stuck in a cycle of judging, criticising, analysing, blaming and diagnosing myself. My attention was not on myself, or what I could do to change. I felt I could 'do' no more. I felt overwhelmed, disempowered and fatigued. I had run out of ideas. If anyone had told me then that there was something I could do that would make a difference, I would have laughed out loud. How could one person make a difference in such a monolithic bureaucracy? As far as I was concerned, it was the system that was wrong, and the bullying that is part of that system.

The years up to and after publication of *The Bullying Culture* (Hadikin and O'Driscoll, 2000) have led me to look at solutions. I could not avoid the fact that the 'system' is made up of people like us. You and me. People make the system and every one of us has a part to play. In writing *The Bullying Culture,* we identified coaching as a possible solution, but minimised the potential of coaching because back then we could hardly see it ourselves. Coaching was new and we were uncertain what, if any, effect it could have. Since then, and since working as a coach with many people on both sides of the bully-victim dyad, I have come to realise the potential for coaching is monumental. Coaching has the potential to turn around the culture of the NHS, as it has in other organisations, and it begins with us. We can make a difference by turning our attention to ourselves.

This is not to minimise the difficulties of working within a bullying culture. The culture is real, and its effects have serious implications for our health (Hadikin and O'Driscoll, 2000). In addition to acknowledging the difficulties, we need also to realise that we have enormous power to change, power that we are not yet acknowledging. Just as bullying is a negative interaction, an immature way of communicating, so coaching is a positive interaction and a mature way of communicating. The negative effects of a bullying culture can be ameliorated, if not reversed, by developing a coaching culture (Hadikin, 2002). Each of us has the power to begin this change right now by paying attention to our thoughts, words, feelings, and by paying attention to who we are being when we show up for work and who we are being in our interactions with our colleagues. Self-awareness is the first step to raising our EQ and we obtain this awareness through self-observation. The effects of coaching are not limited to the individual being coached; rather, they ripple out way beyond the individual being coached to permeate departments and the whole organisation. The coaching effect is contagious.

Coaching enables us to build a strong personal foundation, set personal boundaries, prioritise our health and wellbeing, and develop a strong sense of self.

A STRONG PERSONAL FOUNDATION

If the foundation is strong, a building will last many, many years and withstand repairs and upgrades. If a building has shaky foundations, it will be unstable no matter how much work we put into repairing and maintaining it. What does having a strong personal foundation mean to us? If we have a strong foundation it means we have stability. Something to build the rest of our lives upon. On a practical level, this means identifying our personal needs and taking steps to ensure they are met. This also means putting structures in place to ensure they are met permanently, so that we have a sense of security.

Having a strong personal foundation means building reserves of as many resources as possible, to support us through difficult times. Normally we tend to think of resources in a rather limited way, such as finances. Yet resources can also be health, fitness, people, education and EQ. We build reserves in health, by keeping ourselves as fit as possible for our age and ability, aiming for optimum health at all times. We build financial reserves, by ensuring that we clear and avoid debt and always save a percentage of our income, no matter how little that may be. We build our reserves in education by acknowledging our need for growth and committing ourselves to lifelong learning. This gives us the flexibility to adapt to changing circumstances.

We build a reserve of people, by having a supportive network and maintaining our network so that people are there for us when we need them. In addition to having a supporting network, we build our reserve of EQ through developing our relationships with people. Raising our EQ improves our effectiveness in relationship building which, in turn, improves our ability to grow supportive networks for ourselves. This, in turn, raises our EQ even further. Of crucial importance in developing our network is our ability to build relationships before we actually need them.

A middle performer at Bell labs talked about being stumped by a technical problem. He painstakingly called various technical gurus and then waited, wasting valuable time while calls went unreturned and e-mail messages unanswered. Star performers, however, rarely face such situations because they do the work of building reliable networks before they actually need them. When they call someone for advice, stars almost always get a faster answer.

(Kelley and Caplan, 1993)

Coaching Case Study

Debbie is a newly qualified midwife. She has been working on rotation through a postnatal ward and labour suite, and has recently begun working on an antenatal ward. She qualified as a 'direct-entry' midwife and says she is confident and competent in 'normal' midwifery. Since starting on the antenatal ward, however, her confidence has dipped and she says that she is 'out of her depth'. She believes her training prepared her well to be an extremely competent practitioner of normal midwifery – but the women on the antenatal ward do not fit into that category. Mostly they have been admitted to hospital because they have complicated pregnancies and/or medical conditions. Debbie is not qualified as a nurse and feels inadequate in caring for such cases which she admits frighten her. She dreads things going wrong and feels incompetent. She says that every day she feels that a mistake is 'just waiting to happen'. She has informed senior staff of the areas in which she feels she lacks competence, but the ward is short staffed and she often feels 'drawn' into things because no one else is around or available. Debbie came to coaching to build her confidence.

Following coaching, Debbie had much greater clarity about her defined role and competencies. She focused her attention on setting up strong personal boundaries which enabled her to focus her practice on her areas of competence and avoid straying into areas in which she is incompetent. Part of this was learning to admit to her areas of incompetence. Of course we are incompetent. We must be able to acknowledge and respect our incompetence as much as our competence, or we may be tempted to stray into dangerous territory. Knowing where we are incompetent makes us safe practitioners.

When we become uncomfortable it is a sign that we might need to raise our personal standards around an issue. Rather than tolerating our discomfort, we can take the opportunity to clarify our position on the issue and raise our standards. How do we do this? As with anything important we do it gradually and in stages. The first question to ask ourselves is: 'What am I tolerating?'

EXERCISE

Allow 20-30 minutes for the following exercise.

STEP 1

Take a piece of paper and at the top write: 'What am I tolerating?' Divide your sheet into 3 columns. In the first column, writing as quickly as you can, list 100 'tolerations'. Take no longer than 10 minutes. Tolerations are anything that makes you cringe or squirm, anything that makes you uncomfortable, angry, depressed, worried and/or scared. Anything that has been driving you mad, and you have simply put up with it. This can range from the dripping tap in your bathroom to the leaky guttering; or from your husband cutting his toenails at the kitchen table to your manager criticising your work or you not getting your breaks. Anything.

STEP 2
The heading for column 2 is 'Action'. In column 2, adjacent to each toleration in column 1, write what action would need to be taken to remove it permanently from your life. Take into account what resources you need and how long it will take before proceeding to the next step.

STEP 3
The heading for column 3 is 'Date'. In column 3 write the date by which you know your action will be completed. Where you once had tolerations you now have an action plan and a timescale. It is up to you to choose which issues to deal with first. You may choose to deal with a few smaller ones to feel a sense of accomplishment and freedom or you may choose to deal with a big one that is draining you. It is enormously uplifting to rid yourself of irritations.

(I am keen to hear your experience of this exercise. If you are willing, please e-mail your feedback to ruth@dreamcoach.co.uk)

A 'toleration' is a call to raise our standards in a particular area. Having identified what we tolerate, our next step is to create a new standard for ourselves which we express in a 'standard statement'. If, for example, we have been tolerating a colleague's bad language then we might create a standard statement for ourselves which says: 'I do not tolerate bad language'. We do not need to write this down anywhere, except maybe in our coaching or reflective journal. It is simply for our own benefit, so that we gain clarity over the areas where we feel uncomfortable. This is an important step in developing self-awareness.

Before we can have strong personal boundaries we need to know what it is we want to put a boundary around. We have personal boundaries to protect our personal standards. We do not need anyone else's permission or approval. Our standards are about us. If we are tolerating something, and feeling uncomfortable about it, then we are operating beneath our own personal standards. It is not about anybody else. It is about us.

At some time or another we have all experienced working with someone who has higher personal standards than our own. Consider someone who always ensures they are off work on time, and never misses a meal break. We may admire their perceived 'strength' – and yet we may also feel uncomfortable because we are reminded of our own perceived inadequacies. The key word in that sentence is 'perceived'. In reality, the person with high standards is no stronger than anyone else, and a person with low standards and/or weak boundaries is not essentially 'weaker' than anyone else. Developing high standards and strong personal boundaries is simply a skill which we can all learn and it is an important tool for raising our EQ.

Once we have identified a 'toleration' and created our new standard, the next step is to put a boundary around it. Personal boundaries are not barriers between us and others – rather, they are a protection that enables us to be with others without suffering any ill effects from their behaviour. Boundaries enable us to be with others without lowering our standards. They protect our mind, body, soul and emotions.

Strong personal boundaries

In the above coaching case study, Debbie worked on setting higher professional standards for herself. She undertook some fieldwork, by sitting down and drawing up a list of professional standards that were important to her. She listed her professional values, and identified where she felt her practice was out of alignment with them. In doing so she also identified specifically where she felt competent, partly competent or incompetent. Once she had this information she became much clearer about what she was and was not willing to undertake in her role. It still took tremendous courage for her to return to her workplace and implement her new standards. She still needed strong boundaries to protect her standards and to ensure that she did not stray into areas where she felt uncomfortable.

Once we have raised our standards, it is important that we confirm our commitment by telling someone. In Debbie's case, discussing this with her coach and her Supervisor of Midwives was an important step. She informed an appropriate authority of the areas in which she was not competent to practice. She requested extra tuition in some areas. Her Supervisor was impressed by her professionalism and by the responsible way she handled herself.

Once Debbie had identified her standards, the challenge was to maintain them. Debbie found circumstances were difficult and, as a newly qualified midwife within her first year of professional practice, she often felt overwhelmed by her responsibilities. Telling people helped. She found that the senior midwives were much more helpful than she had imagined. Once everyone knew

Debbie's level of practice they were less likely to leave her in situations where she felt ill at ease.

SIX STAGES OF BOUNDARY SETTING

Appropriate language helps us to assert our boundaries effectively. Our language should always reflect that the boundary is about us and not the other person. It is our discomfort, our standard and our boundary. It really is never about the other person. We therefore avoid accusations which may trigger a defensive response in others. To set our boundaries effectively, we want the other person to co-operate with us. To achieve this we avoid statements which attack the other person, call them names or make them 'wrong' in any way.

An example of poor boundary setting may be: 'You are making me feel sick lighting that cigarette while I'm eating. You are just so selfish.'

In the above example we have accused the other person of something ('You are making me feel sick') and we have extended our accusation to diagnose them as a 'bad person' ('You are just so selfish'). They are likely to feel attacked and to become defensive. As they are preparing their defence, they are probably not listening, and nothing has altered the status quo. They will probably continue to smoke, and we will continue to feel sick.

An example of good boundary setting is: 'Do you know that cigarette smoke is making me feel sick?'

This is much better. It simply presents the other person with the information without accusations or making them 'wrong' in any way. We offer simple information about us. Remember: boundaries are always about us. We can never be certain what another person is thinking, so we keep the focus on ourselves and keep a neutral tone of voice without an emotional charge (see charge neutral, Chapter 3).

Inform

The first stage in setting our boundaries is to simply inform the person of our new standard. As in the above example, we simply give information about us, in a charge neutral tone of voice, and without accusation. Then be quiet. Allow the other person room to respond. Do not over explain or justify your standard. The more you can keep it about how you feel, the better. For example: 'Do you know that I felt uncomfortable when you questioned me in front of that client?'

It is really difficult for anyone to argue with this. How would they know how you felt? They can hardly say: 'No, you didn't.'

A great opener is the phrase: 'Do you know...?' At this stage, remember, we are simply informing them.

Request

Many people will change their behaviour after you have simply informed them. If they do not, you may desire to move to the next stage and make a request. Again, keep it short and to the point. For example: 'I request that you not question my practice in front of clients.'

Educate

This is where you have the opportunity to offer an alternative way. The other person may genuinely not know any way to be, other than to continue doing what they have always done. If they still step over your boundaries, offer a new way forward. For example: 'When you have need to question my actions, could we do this in the office?'

Warn

The first three stages are gentle prompts and guides. After this, you may need to become firmer if someone is particularly intransigent. It is time to warn them that you are no longer willing to tolerate such behaviour. For example: 'I warn you that I am not willing to tolerate your questioning me in front of clients.'

Demand

This is where you take a firmer stand for yourself. For example: 'I have told you how I feel about this, and I demand that you respect my wishes by not questioning me again in front of a client.'

Note that your language is becoming stronger and firmer to reflect your commitment to taking a stand to protect your boundaries.

Leave

If the other person has not changed their behaviour, it is up to you to prove that you really mean it and that you really will not tolerate their behaviour. Your language should be firm but open to discussion at some future date. For example: 'You obviously do not respect my wishes. I am willing to discuss this with you at a future date but at this moment I am leaving.'

You must walk away, leave the room, and demonstrate a firm commitment to your own boundaries.

Boundary setting is not easy. It takes courage, commitment, patience, practice and persistence. Other people will test you to see whether you 'really mean it'. They will have 'change back' reactions. You must prepare yourself for this, and be prepared to ride it out. This is where having a coach can help you to stay clear about your boundaries and focused on your goal.

NOT IN FRONT OF THE CHILDREN...

We have seen how to deal with issues when they arise, but a common factor for many practitioners is that this is often in front of a client, and it seems unprofessional to challenge a colleague in front of them. Even in our homes we feel uncomfortable about discussing important issues in front of our children. Why do we avoid standing up for ourselves in front of others? Is it because we believe we are protecting our clients (and our children)? Yet at the same time we are depriving them of a valuable opportunity to witness, and learn, advanced emotional literacy.

When we become emotionally literate, confident and competent in our interpersonal skills, it is worth considering whether to assert our boundaries in front of our clients and children so that we become role models for them. How are they to develop emotional literacy if they never witness it? As we become skilled in EQ ourselves we become role models for others.

This is a common situation for professionals. I once had three clients experience this dilemma within the same week. One was a teacher, one a midwife, and one a manager. In all three cases they received verbal abuse from a colleague. Each one felt they had good reason to not challenge their 'abuser' at the time because they felt it was 'unprofessional' to do so. (Note that in all three cases the 'abuser' did not stop to think that their behaviour was unprofessional before verbally abusing them in front of their clients.) Yet putting it off gave the impression to the abuser that their behaviour was condoned. It also sent a message to the witness that this behaviour is acceptable and goes unchallenged. The witnesses were deprived of a wonderful opportunity to learn how they could handle such a situation when it happens to them at some stage in their life. Everyone missed an opportunity to raise their EQ. We cannot raise our EQ by avoiding the emotional 'classroom'. Every human relationship offers us an opportunity to raise our EQ: to learn to do something differently, to learn to do something better.

It takes courage to be coached

I know from personal experience that it takes courage to be a coachee. When I began working with my first coach I felt very vulnerable. I worked with her on unravelling why I was not achieving what I wanted to. We examined my stumbling blocks; looked at my bad habits; identified ways I sabotage myself and uncovered the 'stories' I was telling myself to explain why I was not more successful. All my 'failings' were set out before me. There was no hiding place. It took a lot of courage to accept this and to trust that someone was sincere in her intention to help me and really was not judging me. I had become cynical. It took courage, and a willingness to be open to new ways of being, to change this.

EQ and conflict resolution

Emotional intelligence helps in conflict resolution within our social groups – not just in the workplace, but at home too. On many occasions we negotiate, analyse the social situation, organise others, lead and model skills for others. When conflict arises between group members, we may help to resolve conflict by demonstrating advanced emotional skills. Imagine a heated family argument where one or more members of the family have the ability to remain calm and objective. Imagine having the opportunity to discuss what happened with another member of the family. Imagine the whole family becoming aware of family behaviour patterns. Imagine the effective use of questions within your family such as: 'How could you have done it differently?'

Imagine breaking away from an apparently hereditary behaviour such as chronic worrying. As we develop our self-awareness, we become aware of our own thought patterns and how to change them. We notice when our thinking is likely to be depressogenic (causing depression). As we work with a coach, we become skilled at changing our thoughts, and therefore our beliefs about ourselves. We challenge our own negativity, our limiting beliefs and our negative self-talk, and at the same time acknowledge our strengths. We can break free from the worry cycle.

BREAKING THE WORRY CYCLE

Worrying is negative daydreaming in which our undisciplined minds habitually run through a sequence of increasingly negative scenarios. In a completely undisciplined stream of consciousness we allow our minds to wander through an increasingly worsening series of worst-case scenarios: each more disastrous than the last. This increases our fear, anxiety, indolence, pessimism and reinforces negative self-belief. Our minds jump from one negative 'What if?' to another, until we become so anxious that we give up our plans or goals.

EXERCISE

The worry cycle can be halted and reversed with this exercise. The technique is simple but requires patience and persistence. First, a degree of self-awareness is necessary to notice the negative train of thought in its infancy. Then we take steps to effectively derail the negative thoughts.

Step 1: Be fully present in the moment
Take note of the present moment: Where are you? What time is it? What are you doing? Look around the room and remind yourself of something you love.

Step 2. Replace negative thoughts with positive ones
Imagine your best case scenario. It may be the case that we dare not even dream that the best case scenario will happen. We fear 'building our hopes up' and so we give ourselves permission to believe the worst will happen, but not the best. We will not even allow ourselves to imagine it. Yet by letting go of our fear of 'false hope', and replacing the negative thought flow with a positive thought flow, we focus our attention in a positive way. Use your imagination to create increasingly 'best' case scenarios. Have fun with this. Allow yourself to envision the best, then build on it until it is better. Then practice your 'visioning' every day, making it better each time. Never fear 'false hope'. Hope never hurt anyone.

(I am keen to hear your experience of this exercise. If you are willing, please e-mail your feedback to ruth@dreamcoach.co.uk)

By stopping the negative stream of thought and replacing it with a positive one, hope and optimism, rather than fear and pessimism, become the habitual train of thought. We break the worry habit and our thoughts habitually become more positive and lighter. This has beneficial effects on our health and on our performance. We are lighter, more inspired, more creative, and more likely to come up with creative solutions to our problems when an optimistic outlook prevails. We experience an 'attitude' shift, from 'There's no way around it, so there's no point in trying' to 'There must be a way around this'. Through trying and experimenting we may discover a solution, but first we must be open to the possibility.

FEAR

Overcoming fear is probably one of our greatest challenges. Consider what you would do in your life if you had no fear whatsoever. Part of our journey to greater self-awareness is acknowledging our fear. Fear is natural and is part of our inborn mechanism of self-protection (see Chapter 2). We fear unfamiliar situations and change. If we only ever stayed within the boundaries of the safe and familiar, we could never come to any harm. We would never do anything different in our lives either. Sometimes to live life to the full we must learn to overcome our natural fear and resistance. This means recognising where fear holds us back, and where we allow fear to sabotage our plans.

In developing a greater sense of self, and becoming more self-aware, we develop a greater sense of self-preservation. This means we may initially experience greater fear and anxiety, and this can be beneficial. This increased fear and anxiety is what alerts us to danger and gives us the opportunity to make different choices. This can even save our lives. Birmingham postal worker Jermaine Lee committed suicide following prolonged workplace bullying (Hadikin, 2002). Had he made different choices he might still be alive today. The choices he made kept him in a situation that was physically and psychologically damaging him. The key is to acknowledge our fear and to understand what it is about. In some situations we suppress important feelings, perhaps telling ourselves we are being 'illogical', when in fact an acknowledgement of our feelings could alert us to a safer course of action or at least one that is more appropriate for our needs.

Once we become more self-aware, we develop our ability to distinguish between those fears which will protect us and those which are impeding our growth.

In self-preservation it is most important to develop awareness of where we have choices and what our options are. Noticing our thoughts, and paying attention to them, are the first steps to consciously lift our own moods.

WHY WOULD YOU HIRE YOUR OWN COACH?

We have seen how working with a coach could help you to:

- become a masterful communicator
- be a role model for others
- be influential in your workplace
- be someone who others listen to
- be a leader
- be a coach, mentor or preceptor
- raise your EQ
- empower yourself
- feel in control of how you experience your life and work
- develop your sense of self
- manage your self better
- have personal space and time
- balance work and home life
- enjoy your life and work
- be someone who takes initiative
- be more effective – both personally and professionally
- have a supportive and energising personal and professional network: be surrounded by people who inspire, support and energise you, and
- improve the quality of your personal and professional relationships.

In future, coaching may be readily available through a network of peers who are trained and experienced in coaching skills. Until such time arrives, we may choose to experience coaching by hiring a personal coach for a period of time to enable us to jump-start our EQ. Do you have access to a coach in your workplace? If so, are your coaching sessions scheduled to take place regularly, or are you coached on an *ad hoc* basis? Do you have a choice of coach?

The next chapter discusses how you can apply coaching skills within a healthcare setting and effectively coach your clients. Before attempting this, it is advisable to avail yourself of some quality coaching and experience being a coachee first-hand. If you are interested in having access to coaching, and there is no formal coaching support available in your workplace yet, you could hire a personal coach or you could set up a coaching circle in your workplace where you and your colleagues peer coach one another. There is more information on setting up coaching circles later in this book. You can now refer to the coach directory at the back of this book to generate a shortlist of personal coaches who will be happy to discuss their coaching style with you and to explore how coaching could benefit you personally.

This chapter opened with a quote from Ghandi: 'Each of us must be the change we want to see in the world.' Ghandi meant that we must embrace the very qualities we wish to see more of in the world; so, for example, if we want to live in a peaceful world we must live peacefully. Likewise, if we want to live and work in a nurturing, coaching culture, rather than a bullying culture, we must learn to become nurturing coaches and be willing to be coached.

5

Being the coach: the coach practitioner

Let us be grateful to people who make us happy; they are the charming gardeners who make our souls blossom.
Marcel Proust

We have seen that coaching encompasses a philosophy and a skill set which accelerates and supports the natural human developmental process. The role of the coach is to create a nurturing environment in which the coachee can further their own growth. I often use gardening as an analogy. The seed for our potential already exists within every one of us. Like a gardener, a good coach focuses on creating a nurturing environment in which the coachee blossoms to reach their potential. Also like a gardener, some of our 'plants' might be healthier than others, and through our coaching some may become healed. This is where there is some confusion, because coaching is not therapy and is not solely intended to be therapeutic. Yet sometimes emotional healing does take place, almost as a side-effect, within the context of a coaching relationship. This is not because of any intentional 'cure' applied by the coach but rather as a result of our natural tendency to heal when we are in a nurturing environment. As healthcare practitioners we understand that healing is a natural process which takes place given an optimum environment.

If coaching is a process, a tool, or even a 'style' that we can adopt to generate a nurturing environment, which enables (without directly causing) healing, then it has important implications for healthcare. This chapter will begin to explore how coaching skills and knowledge may be applied to a healthcare setting to bring the nurturing benefits of coaching to our clients. This is nothing new. Healthcare practitioners have always striven to create the optimum environment for healing. Through intentionally structuring coaching sessions, the process of creating this nurturing relationship can be named, acknowledged and applied with intent. In later chapters we will extend this principle to managerial and organisational level so that we may extend this process to generate a nurturing culture of healthcare.

As we have seen, coaching is a philosophy underpinned by an eclectic collection of skills, many of which are congruent with nursing, midwifery, psychotherapeutic and counselling skills. It is therefore possible to adopt a coaching approach to your healthcare practice in whichever field of healthcare that may be. Choosing along the continuum from directive to non-directive coaching you would be able to discern which coaching style is more suited to your particular field of practice and to each particular client situation.

It is also useful for healthcare practitioners, in the context of our own professional development, to be able to identify which of our skills are coaching skills and to possess the ability to use them effectively. Coaching is a valuable skill set which is transferable to many workplace situations outside of healthcare. Coaching gives healthcare practitioners a way to 'package' their skills to potential employers so that non-healthcare managers can understand the skill set involved. Coaching is increasingly recognised as a valuable asset in every manager's toolbox, so when applying for managerial posts it is worthwhile being able to demonstrate coaching skills and experience.

Examples of coaching interventions in healthcare practice are, at the time of writing, still relatively rare although there is some documented evidence. Examples of coaching interventions can be found in various fields of healthcare: Whittemore, Chase, Mandle and Roy (2001) examined the effects of nurse coaching interventions in Type 2 diabetes, whilst Vale and colleagues demonstrated that patients with coronary heart disease who received telephone coaching had significantly lower cholesterol after six months than those not coached, and that more coached patients actually reached the target level than those not coached (Vale et al, 2002). Research is also being designed to monitor the effect of telephone coaching (among other factors) in patients with cancer pain. This study group will be monitored for differences in pain intensity, quality of life and functional status (Douglas, 2002). See the 'further reading' section at the end of this book for more documented examples of coaching interventions.

As the paradigm of healthcare shifts towards greater self-management, with more emphasis on personal responsibility, coaching emerges as a potentially effective tool for enabling clients to take responsibility for the management of their condition.

EXERCISE

Before reading on, take some time to consider the following questions and make a note of your responses.

How could coaching benefit your clinical practice?

What difference could it make to you, both personally and in your professional capacity?

What difference could coaching make to clinical outcomes?

How does coaching fit with evidence-based practice?

(I am keen to hear your experience of this exercise. If you are willing, please e-mail your feedback to ruth@dreamcoach.co.uk)

As clients take personal responsibility for their health, the role of healthcare practitioners changes. Coaching clients through a process of healing and transition will play a much larger part in healthcare.

DETACHMENT FROM THE OUTCOME

This was mentioned in Chapter 3 and is worth reviewing here in a little more detail because this can be an especially challenging area for us as healthcare practitioners. We care about our clients. This seems obvious. We would not do what we do otherwise. So how can we not care about the outcome? Detachment does not mean we do not care about our clients – rather, it is a frame of mind where we focus our attention on supporting our clients rather than attaching ourselves to the goal. This means we can continue to offer unconditional support to our client even if they fail to reach their goal.

Clients are responsible for themselves. People will do what they want to do despite our best efforts to change them and, very often, in spite of us. If our clients choose to, they will walk out of our clinic, smoke 40 cigarettes, drink 16 pints of lager and then breastfeed their infant. We may be shocked, dismayed, disappointed, horrified, but we are not responsible for them. In coaching our clients we must detach ourselves from the outcome. This means that we must not 'push' our clients toward a stated objective. When we have no attachment to a specific course of action we are open and flexible in our approach. We are able to discuss various options with our clients and to support their choice. We will continue to nurture our clients' growth without stifling them, so they will feel free to move in any direction they choose. For coaching to be successful it is essential that we learn the art of detaching ourselves from the outcome and respecting our clients' choices. If we appear to be rigidly pushing our clients towards a specific outcome this is not coaching – it may even be a bullying style.

Detachment can be difficult if we are coaching a client toward a specific health objective, for example a blood cholesterol level of less than 5.0 mmol/L. It is all too easy to focus on the goal, rather than on our client, urging them on and pushing them towards the objective. Yet it is precisely this 'pushiness' which may lead our client to give up and to sabotage their own progress. We may push them too fast and run into their resistance. They may begin to feel that we really do not care about them at all, and that we are only interested in achieving the goal. By coaching them through their own experience, encouraging them to observe themselves, to notice where they experience resistance and to notice for themselves when they sabotage their own progress, we send the message that we really care about who they are, and about how they feel. This way they learn so much more about themselves, and learn to be responsible for themselves. We must learn to let go of feeling responsible for them. One client recently said to me: 'You don't care if I reach this goal.' I was pleased that the client had noticed my non-attachment. My reply was: 'I care that you do your best, and I am not attached to the outcome. So you are right. Whilst I care about you, I have no attachment to whether you reach this goal or not. That is up to you.'

Clients are responsible for themselves, as we are responsible for ourselves. Coaching helps us to make a clear distinction between our responsibility to the client, our responsibility for ourselves and our client's responsibility for themselves. When we coach our clients we are helping them to become responsible for themselves by empowering them and helping them to see where they have choices. When we put the client in control we enable her to make decisions about her own care, empowering her, and helping her see where she has power and can make choices. With this power comes responsibility. Once clients become aware of the fact that they have power, and that their choices make a difference, they assume responsibility for themselves and the choices they make.

This has implications in helping to change the current 'blame' culture. Once we make a significant paradigm shift towards personal responsibility, we stop blaming others. We shift our focus from making others responsible for our circumstances and we begin to take control of our own lives.

GROUP COACHING

One of the most powerful uses of coaching is within a group dynamic. Whether we are part of a team within a clinical setting or whether we are part of a team that meets regularly to work on a particular project, coaching can radically improve the performance of the group as a whole. By having a repertoire of coaching skills such as listening and effective questioning, we can move a team forward, whether we have any formal leadership role or not.

Coaching affords us an opportunity to develop and apply our leadership skills. If we have the opportunity to work with groups of clients we can apply our coaching skills within a group setting.

Coaching with a group is not significantly different from one-to-one coaching, although there are different skills involved. It might also be helpful to distinguish between facilitation and group coaching. Facilitation generally focuses on the goals or objectives of the group, team or organisation. Group coaching still focuses on the individual, even though they are part of a group. So with group coaching the individual's growth and development is still paramount. This is not to say that within a group any one individual takes priority, but rather that all the members of the group are able to receive the support that coaching can offer, at the same time. An example in clinical practice may be a group of women who meet regularly for coaching in breastfeeding.

Remember that you already possess many coaching skills. Acknowledging this fact and striving to bring coaching wisdom and skills into your practice will enhance your practice. You will also be able to bring your coaching skills to bear in other fields, should you desire a career change.

So what is it that you do that is coaching? We have seen that coaching is a term that, like nursing or midwifery, encompasses a set of skills and philosophies and offers a number of models or tools through which your skills and philosophy can be presented.

Consider the range of coaching skills outlined in Chapter 3 and note how many you already use in your practice. When you are listening you are coaching. When you are simply being with a client, you are coaching. When you are encouraging them, you are coaching. When your belief in them is greater than their belief in themselves, you are coaching. As mentioned earlier, much of the positive, nurturing side of healthcare is congruent with coaching. You already possess many coaching skills which you probably do not acknowledge as coaching. When you apply these skills in a structured way, with the intention of supporting your clients to achieve specific outcomes, you will be coaching intentionally.

The difference is one of awareness and intention. It is the crucial difference between offering occasional encouragement in the hope that it helps in some way, and offering structured coaching sessions, of which encouragement may be part, in a skilled manner, at the appropriate time, and knowing that it will make a difference to the outcome. Using the gardening analogy again, it is the difference between throwing a few seeds out of the window in the hope that some may grow, and deliberately choosing the best place, preparing the ground and creating the best conditions possible to ensure that they *will* grow. It is the difference between coaching by default and coaching intentionally.

Structuring coaching sessions

If you intend to coach, do it in a structured way and ask the client's permission. Coach consciously, with a full awareness of what you are doing and why. Structuring coaching sessions means setting time aside for the sole purpose of coaching. From the outset, ask the client what the focus of the coaching should be. Remember, you will be working to the client's agenda not your own. You may initially set up six weekly coaching sessions as a follow-up from a course of treatment or to support a client in a new course of treatment. Whatever the reason for the coaching sessions, allow the client to set the agenda right from the start.

This does not mean you abdicate your role as a healthcare professional. Your advice is important and you should let the client know you are willing to be consulted. If possible, give your client a range of options. For example, a client who has been smoking may discuss with her nurse practitioner whether to stop suddenly or to give up gradually, and what is the 'best' way. The nurse practitioner in a coaching role would present the information as a range of options and ask the client to choose a way forward that feels comfortable for them. In the follow-up coaching session the nurse-coach would ask the client to give feedback on their experience of the method they chose and whether they still feel comfortable with it, or whether they would like to modify their approach in some way. The nurse-coach might inquire whether they are happy with their rate of progress: Is it too easy? Or is it too challenging? Are they experiencing resistance? The nurse-coach may simply 'be with' the client as they talk about their experience, good or bad, of giving up smoking.

The coaching focus is on discovering the most appropriate way to support each individual client, given that people are unique individuals and what may motivate one person may demotivate another. Whether the client has achieved their intended goal for the week or not, by listening to the client's experience, the coach will discover valuable information about the issues that this client is experiencing. By sharing this with the client they, in turn, learn valuable information about themselves. Coach and client then co-create a way forward that this client will find slightly challenging but not overwhelming. It is important to achieve the right balance with each individual client so that they stay in the flow state: experiencing the thrill of success without being bored because it is 'too easy' or giving up because it is 'too difficult'.

Positive reinforcement is important, to spur the client on to achieve greater success. When a client has made a significant breakthrough, achieved a goal or objective, or succeeded in only a small way it is important to take some time with them to acknowledge their achievement and, importantly, to encourage them to acknowledge themselves. Some people may wish to rush on to the next success without taking time to appreciate the success they have just achieved. It is important to slow such people down, if only for a moment, to acknowledge them, and to encourage them to 'be with' their own success for a moment.

Invariably such people chase success after success without experiencing much sense of satisfaction or fulfillment from their achievements. Learning to acknowledge themselves can lead to greater fulfillment and a richer experience of coaching for them.

Towards the end of each coaching session, it is helpful to ask the client to evaluate the coaching session itself. This can be simple verbal feedback on what they most valued in the session and what they found of least value. This enables the coach to tailor future coaching sessions to this client's needs.

Finally, the coach should always ask the client what their goals or objectives are in the coming week. The client may set their own or the coach may request that the client meets a specific objective, remembering that the client may not always agree to the coach's request. It is important that some fieldwork is agreed upon, before the end of the coaching session, that will build on the success of last week and move the client forward. There is no failure, since every experience is an opportunity for a learning experience. Even if the client felt that last week was a 'failure', there will be some rich learning in the experience for them if the coach is experienced enough to encourage the client to reflect and observe their own behaviour patterns.

PEER COACHING

How can you begin to put your new-found coaching skills into practice? One way to practice your coaching skills is by coaching your colleagues. Imagine a situation where a colleague comes to you and asks your advice about something. In the past, you might have taken on the role of advice-giver or expert and said 'do it this way' or 'do it that way' – or even offered to do it for them. On this occasion you could choose to take a coaching approach. Even though it is your colleague, and the coaching may be impromptu, you can still ensure the coaching session is structured. You may initiate coaching by saying something like: 'I see your problem, would you like some coaching around this?' With permission, you might then ask your colleague: 'What are the options?'

Listen, and allow your colleague to suggest every option that she can think of. Request that your colleague write them down. Then, add your ideas to the list. Your colleague now has many more options than she originally thought of. Hearing your responses may also spark her imagination so that she envisions options that she had not previously thought of. This may, in turn, inspire you so that you add even more options to the growing list. This is how the synergy of coaching works in practice.

If you are both having fun and approach it lightly you are also likely to generate more ideas than if you felt bogged down by the exercise. This is synergy at work. You co-create something that is greater than what either or both of you could have created by working alone.

If time permits you might, at this point, wish to move the coaching session forward by asking your colleague a question that encourages them to think through some of the options, such as: 'What would be the consequences of each option?'

Alternatively, you could request that your colleague approach this as fieldwork, or you may schedule a follow-up coaching session to discuss it.

If your colleague agrees to your request to do this as fieldwork you would then place it within a timeframe by asking: 'When will you do it?' And then build in accountability by asking: 'How will I know when you've done it?'

We can see that a structured coaching session with a colleague may well be inpromptu, but still contains the essential elements of:

- a synergistic relationship
- goal-setting within a timeframe
- accountability
- commitment, and
- follow-up.

Even if your colleague has chosen to do some fieldwork you can still schedule another chat to follow-up on your coaching session and ask about their progress. This can be done in ten minutes next time you are working together, or as a ten minute 'check-in' over the telephone.

Once you have finished, it is still important to complete your session by drawing attention to the process itself so that your colleague recognises the coaching process and is able to distinguish it from mentoring or counselling. This encourages your colleague to recognise how your coaching facilitates their growth, and to appreciate the value of the coaching. You might want to ask your colleague what value they perceived, if any, from the coaching session. This will provide you with feedback on your own coaching skills. You might want to ask how they felt about coaching, rather than advice giving, as a response to their original question. In effect, you briefly evaluate the coaching session and ask your colleague to give you feedback. All feedback is valuable. If your colleague did not find the coaching session helpful, it is equally important that you understand why. Perhaps the two of you are incompatible, perhaps it was not an appropriate situation for coaching, or perhaps you need to polish your coaching skills a little. If so, which ones? Were you listening well? Did you ask questions? Were you telling your colleague what to do instead of encouraging her to create her own solutions?

The intention in coaching is to assist your colleague in developing her own solutions, responsibility, accountability and proactivity. If you were tempted to give advice which your colleague followed, and then it turned out to be an ineffective choice, she may be left feeling resentful, critical and blaming. Indeed, she may blame you – after all, it was your advice! Advice-giving can actually foster the blame culture, especially between peers. Coaching enhances and encourages empowerment, accountability and autonomy. You might even start a trend. You will certainly notice a difference in your workplace as a culture of coaching slowly evolves.

Another way that you could experience coaching with your colleagues is to set up coaching circles which meet regularly. A coaching circle is a group of like-minded friends or colleagues who agree to meet regularly for the purpose of coaching one another and advancing each other's personal and/or professional development. For a coaching circle to be successful it is important that the members of the group take time to bond and trust one another. This cannot work with different members leaving and joining each week. It may therefore be better to agree to meet regularly, maybe every week, for a fixed period of time, perhaps an eight week period, and the group agree to stay together and not to admit any new members during this time. The group can agree to some ground rules which will facilitate the group and the coaching. These will ultimately be the group's choice and may, for example, include agreements on avoiding negativity. Some groups begin by having a ten minute 'BMW' zone. 'BMW' stands for bitching, moaning and whining. Once the ten minutes is over, the group's attention turns toward creating positive solutions and no more 'BMW' is permitted within the group. Remember that in coaching, the focus is always on the individuals within the group rather than on the group's goals. The group is there to lend support and to offer coaching to the individuals within.

So what makes coaching different from just a brainstorming session? First the intention behind the dialogue. Brainstorming may or may not be part of the coaching session, it depends on whatever the individual coachee's goal is. With coaching, the intent is always to move the coachee forward toward taking some action, or making a decision, in respect of their objective. The second difference is the commitment to taking some action, based on the outcome of the brainstorming. The third difference is the accountability, or follow-up.

It is worth reminding ourselves at this point that the goal of coaching is to help us improve. So the action we choose may actually mean doing less – certainly if we are already overwhelmed and under stress. It is tempting to only think of doing more when we see the word 'action', yet the outcome of a coaching session could quite easily be a commitment to agree to do less, or to change a commitment to which we had previously agreed, if our objective is to create more time and space for ourselves.

Another coaching session may seem more like a counselling session than a brainstorming. Imagine you have a client who is facing a dilemma over a course of treatment. The consequences of both choices may be painful: without treatment, the patient would die, but the treatment is painful, uncomfortable and could result in hair loss. After which they may die anyway. The coaching intention remains the same: to help move the client forward to a place where they can make a choice and be comfortable with their choice. Through coaching you can help a client realise they do have choices where they felt they had none. Through the process of coaching the client becomes clearer about which choices they are most comfortable with. Sometimes we feel overwhelmed by what seems to be a multitude of choices, some of which our family and friends think we should make, and others which appeal to us, but that we know family members or our friends, colleagues or partners may not support. It is difficult for us to decide what to do for the best. In coaching, we encourage clients to be true to themselves which often means an exploration into who the 'self' actually is.

Even where a situation appears dire or hopeless, we still have choices. We have a choice about how to react or respond to our circumstances. This point was highlighted by Victor Frankl (1997) a survivor of Auschwitz and other death camps in Nazi Germany. Frankl recognised that, despite imprisonment, starvation and torture, he had freedom. His freedom lay in the gap between stimulus and response. He realised that only he had the power to choose his response to whatever circumstances he found himself in, and therein lay his freedom. Frankl recognised that no one, neither the Nazis nor anyone else, could take this freedom away. He was the only one who had this power. Through this knowledge, he became empowered. Through this same knowledge, we empower ourselves, our clients and our colleagues. No matter how dire our circumstances, we always have a choice. It is the coach's role to cast enough light onto a situation to enable us to begin to see what our choices might be.

6

The coach manager

Coaching offers personal control. A primary cause of stress in the workplace is lack of personal control.

Sir John Whitmore (1996)

Whether you are in clinical practice, a management role, or both, coaching skills are a useful addition to your skills toolbox. What does being a coach manager mean? It may be that coaching is a formalised part of your role, explicit or implicit in your job description, or coaching may simply be a managerial style which you choose to adopt. Either way, you can be a coach manager. In today's stressful working environment, where we are increasingly exhorted to achieve better results with fewer resources, why would you want to add something more to your plate if you do not need to? Because if you have a managerial aspect to your role, if you are responsible for other people, then coaching will undoubtedly make your life easier and reduce stress in your area of responsibility.

Research presented [by Dr Mark Van Vugt from Southampton University] at the British Psychological Society has demonstrated that an oppressive leadership style can result in group members wanting to leave, potentially causing a group to collapse. Given a democratic leadership style, they are more likely to want to stay and help their group. These effects have implications for managers and politicians who are concerned about such issues as employee turnover and the 'brain drain'.

(Internet document: http://www.hrzone.co.uk/item/75209 accessed March 27, 2002)

So, as a manager, how will coaching benefit you directly?

- Coaching will increase responsibility in those for whom you are responsible.

- Coaching will make it easier for you to delegate.
- Coaching will encourage your staff to create solutions rather than come to you with problems expecting you to have all the answers.
- Coaching will reduce stress and generate a healthier working environment. This alone will reduce staff turnover, reduce the costly effects of workplace bullying and improve the sickness/absence figures.

If you are responsible for staff, even just one or two, and you have not yet discovered the benefits of coaching then, for you, this could be the most important chapter in this book.

It is not my intention to repeat how to coach staff. This information has been covered in depth in Chapter 3 and, in this case, the 'coachee' will be a member of staff. It is more important for those of us with a managerial role to understand the benefits of adopting a coach manager style.

REDUCING WORKPLACE STRESS

Many core services are associated with extremely stressful working environments. These include delivery suites, operating theatres, intensive and special care units, coronary care units, accident and emergency departments, not to mention 'first on the scene' paramedic and ambulance services. This list is not exhaustive and in the field of healthcare there are many more. It is, indeed, the nature of the work. This is no excuse for not making every effort to reduce stress, and to support the staff within these areas. Staff support is variable throughout the health service and is better in some areas than others. At the time of writing, in the UK there are still regions where front-line paramedics, and other emergency service employees such as police and fire officers, are regularly exposed to horrific scenes with no debriefing, post-trauma counselling or support services at all. If you are a manager responsible for people in any of the aforementioned areas you can make an immediate difference to stress levels in your ward or department by adopting a coach manager style. I am not suggesting you become a staff counsellor. As you read on through this chapter you will see how changing your managerial style by adopting a coaching approach can greatly reduce stress and encourage proactivity in your staff.

In researching *The Bullying Culture* (Hadikin and O'Driscoll, 2000) we noted that the deadliest cause of workplace stress was high pressure combined with low control. This factor alone is responsible for increased mental strain, anxiety, increased blood pressure and greater risk of heart disease. When it is prolonged over time, staff develop chronic mental and physical illness. As a coach manager you have the power to remove one of these factors by increasing personal control.

This increase in personal control happens as a result of the climate of affirmative inquiry that is generated through the coaching process. It is understandable that, when under pressure (bearing in mind that as managers we also feel the pressure) we may resort to instructing or advising when staff ask us what to do. It is sometimes more expedient to respond by telling them to do this or that. Yet this can quickly become a habit and before long we may find that we have fallen into the role of autocratic manager. Our staff give up looking for their own answers and we feel under increasing pressure to tell them what to do all the time. Have you ever felt that no one around you seems to know what to do without asking you? If so, you may have fallen into this trap. Adopting a coaching approach could be a refreshing change for you, and for your staff.

Whitmore (1996) offers a simple acronym which can be adopted to remind busy managers to coach, rather than instruct. Simply remember to GROW your staff:

Goals
Reality
Options
Will.

This simple reminder of the coaching process guides you towards appropriate questions to ask your coachee which encourage them to generate a solution. For example, a member of staff may approach you with a problem. Instead of telling them what to do you use the G-R-O-W acronym to prompt you:

G – prompts you to ask them what goals and/or objectives they are trying to achieve.
R – reminds you to ask them to take a reality check. Are their goals achievable? Do they have the resources they need?
O – reminds you to help them explore their options. You may

offer a brainstorming session and help generate more options than either of you could have done alone.

W – reminds you to ask what action they will commit to, setting it in a timeframe and requesting follow-up.

For coaching to be effective, we need to create a synergistic relationship between equals. You may not have equal rank formally, within the organisational hierarchy, but you can generate a climate of mutual respect for one another as human beings. Remember to treat your staff member with unconditional positive regard and to let go of your attachment to the outcome. It is important, in encouraging personal responsibility, that you allow your coachee genuine ownership of the result, whether it is considered a success or not. Either way, support them for their efforts. Finally, remember to acknowledge their contribution and their level of commitment, and appreciate them and their work.

Acknowledging

For any coach, learning how to acknowledge our coachees is an essential component of the coaching toolbox. For the coach manager, learning how to acknowledge your staff may be one of the most powerful things you ever do. The changes within your unit or department can be phenomenal and will not cost a penny. All it takes is a shift of perspective and a little courage on your part.

Affirmative inquiry

Coaching in management embraces a process of applied affirmative inquiry (sometimes also known as appreciative inquiry). This is another term which derives from American English where the term 'affirmative' means favourable. In the UK we probably associate an inquiry more commonly with an investigation into something that has gone wrong, and we may have negative associations with the term. Affirmative inquiry is a positive process of questioning to affirm, or confirm, that what we are doing is effective. Coaching focuses on what works, so we want to turn our attention to building on our strengths, rather than focusing on what does not work, or on our weaknesses. This affirmative inquiry process also reminds us to appreciate what we already do well. In this way we add value to ourselves and to the service we provide.

In financial terminology, when something decreases in value it is depreciated. When something increases in value it is appreciated. If we want to increase the value of something we need to appreciate it.

When you appreciate something, you ADD value to it by simply appreciating it. When you depreciate something you diminish its value. Unfortunately for us, through [what] the media (and perhaps even a large part of our society) [may want us to believe at times], we exist in a culture that rips everything apart, diminishes it and values nothing.

(Nagy, 2001)

A coach manager can foster a culture of affirmative inquiry by asking questions such as:

What are we doing that works?

What do we do excellently in this unit or department?

Where do we excel above others?

How can we do more of this?

What do you love about this department?

What do we do really well?

What do you do really well?

What are your strengths?

and by encouraging staff to ask similar questions of themselves and their peers.

Strengths-based management

A coach manager will also invest time in identifying people's strengths and ensuring they are employed appropriately. It is inefficient to have someone employed in a position where she is struggling to keep up and barely manages to compensate for her weaknesses. Far better to employ her in a capacity in which she can use her strengths every day. It is also more likely that, in such a role, she will be able to achieve and maintain a 'flow state'. I do not mean a transfer to another field or department – simply allow her to perform those skills which she performs excellently and avoid those which she does not. If each member of staff for whom you are responsible is able to fully utilise their strengths, the overall quality and performance of your department will rise exponentially.

A large-scale survey of 7,939 business units, within 36 companies, suggested that organisations that capitalise on their employees' strengths have lower staff turnover, more productive business units and higher customer satisfaction scores (Buckingham and Clifton, 2002). Why should the health service care about increased productivity? Because we are under pressure to do more, with fewer resources. Why should the health service care about higher customer satisfaction scores? Because, as a general rule, satisfied customers do not sue us. The same survey asked 198,000 employees: 'At work, do you have the opportunity to do what you do best every day?'

The result was 20%. This means that only 20% of employees have the opportunity to utilise their strengths, which means that many organisations are operating at 20% capacity. By discovering and capitalising on your people's strengths there is the potential to improve performance by 80%. I recall working at one time with a consultant anaesthetist who was absolutely abysmal at siting intravenous lines. Yet so much time was wasted, on busy operating days, let alone in an emergency, while everyone politely waited on his sixth, seventh, or even eighth attempt. No one felt they could say or do anything.

We noted in Chapter 2 that Buckingham and Clifton (2002) define a strength as: 'consistent near perfect performance in an activity'. Imagine a culture in which this anaesthetist could fully utilise his strengths whilst delegating this aspect of his role to another anaesthetist, who has 'consistent near perfect performance' in siting intravenous lines. Imagine how much time would be saved. Imagine how many fewer patients would be distressed by his repeated failed attempts. Imagine everyone's confidence restored, including his own, as he develops strengths in other areas and no longer needs to waste time trying to overcome his weakness. Imagine a culture in which he would not feel obliged to struggle and overcome his weaknesses in the first instance. Imagine everyone's overall job satisfaction levels as they are free to concentrate their efforts in areas in which they are confident, skilled and competent.

One of the biggest wastes of time, money and energy I have ever experienced was when I was a Community Midwife. Community Midwives all over the UK are familiar with the annual so-called 'updating' which requires that they spend about two weeks on delivery suite working with core staff, in a hospital unit, 'updating' their core skills. This causes stress for all the midwives involved and bears no relation to their everyday work. Spending two weeks of the year learning procedures related to complicated and abnormal pregnancies, which are outside their level of competence and hence their professional sphere, bears no relation to their role and is no help whatsoever when they next attend a home birth. Yet (at the time of writing) this practice continues to waste midwives' time and taxpayers' money. Studying abnormal labour and complicated pregnancy does not 'update' a Community Midwife in the area of healthy pregnancy and birth.

Guided by the belief that good is the opposite of bad, mankind has for centuries pursued its fixation with fault and failing. Doctors have studied disease in order to learn about health. Psychologists have investigated sadness in order to learn about joy. Therapists have looked into the causes of divorce in order to learn about happy marriage. And in schools and workplaces around the world, each one of us has been encouraged to identify, analyze, and correct our weaknesses in order to become strong.

This advice is well intended but misguided. Faults and failings deserve study, but they reveal little about strengths. Strengths have their own patterns.

To excel in your chosen field and to find lasting satisfaction in doing so, you will need to understand your unique patterns.

(Buckingham and Clifton, 2002)

Of course, in order to be comfortable with subordinates who are excelling themselves, developing their strengths and acquiring a unique sense of self, we have to have a taste of this ourselves. If we do not, if we feel stuck whilst others are forging ahead, we may become jealous, mean-spirited and petty. Jealousy is an interesting concept and worth a brief mention here. When we feel jealous it is because we have recognised in someone, something that we could do ourselves. How often do we experience jealousy and think to ourselves: 'I could have done that'? This is probably because it is true. Envy is natural. Envy is what motivates toddlers to reach up for toys which they can see the bigger children can already reach. Envy encourages us to reach higher. Envy becomes jealousy when we do not try, and we become jealous of those who do. If we are feeling jealous we need to ask ourselves where we have become stuck in our own growth and what do we intend to do about it. This is why I assert that in order to be a great coach we need first to have experienced great coaching.

The hunger for coaching has resulted in hastily and inadequately trained managers, or so-called coaches, failing to meet the expectations of those they are coaching. In too many cases they have not fully understood the performance-related, psychological principles on which coaching is based.

(Whitmore, 1996)

Role models

Great role models for EQ are unfortunately rare in the medical professions. In researching this book I spoke with Dr Ron Arndt, who specialises in coaching dentists. He trained as a dentist himself in the 1970s. He described his training as 'humiliating', and said that he was 'treated like dirt on a good day'.

Two key factors which Dr Arndt has noticed about his clients' dental practices are that many have an extremely high staff turnover, and that his clients do not know how to acknowledge their team. We need role models in our lives. We act as we see. If we have never experienced excellence in EQ we cannot model it for others. According to Dr Arndt, dentists are:

- *time-pressured*
- *broke*
- *constantly in a rat race (like a gerbil in a wheel)*
- *have no business training*
- *underutilize their people skills*
- *do not know how to acknowledge a team*
- *do not have business plans*
- *have not thought strategically for the year ahead*
- *have no annual goal-planning meetings (because they have no annual goals or objectives).*

(Dr Arndt can be found online at www.drarndt.com.)

This implies lack of skill in certain key areas: self-management, communication, financial management, EQ, planning and organisational ability. Emotional intelligence (EQ) is discussed in detail in Chapter 2 – however, it may be worth reminding ourselves at this point of the key factors which contribute to EQ.

A person with greater EQ is able to demonstrate a proficient or advanced level of skill in three specific areas:

- self-awareness
- emotional control, and
- interpersonal skills.

Medical training in the UK has changed over the years to begin to address some of these shortfalls in EQ, yet coaching can still be beneficial. Coaching is based on mutual respect, unconditional positive regard, and the philosophy that the coachee has the answers. This means that it is possible to coach in any direction: up, down or sideways within the managerial hierarchy of the health service. It is therefore possible for a coach manager within a clinical setting, or indeed a practice manager, to be a role model for medical staff in many of the key areas of EQ and to offer coaching in the skills involved.

EXERCISE

Before reading on, take some time to consider the following questions and note your answers.

What difference would coaching make to your professional development?

How would you measure your own 'results'?

How would you measure 'results' in your staff?

How would you monitor your own 'performance'?

How would you monitor the 'performance' of your staff?

What difference would coaching make to your existing managerial style?

What EQ skills can you identify in yourself?

How would you rate your own EQ?

Score yourself on self-awareness, interpersonal skills and emotional control.

Are you: a novice, proficient, an expert, or a master in EQ?

(I am keen to hear your experience of this exercise. If you are willing, please e-mail your feedback to ruth@dreamcoach.co.uk)

Just as coaching is an effective tool for helping patients take responsibility, so coaching as a management style encourages staff to take responsibility for themselves and their professional decisions. I want to introduce the idea of responsibility without blame at this point. All too often the word responsibility carries negative connotations, especially within a climate of fear, bullying, mistrust and blame. Within the blame culture, 'taking responsibility' is often synonymous with finding someone to blame. In the context of coaching, the term 'accepting responsibility' becomes a positive paradigm shift towards acting responsibly and, rather than disempowering us, it has the opposite effect. We feel empowered and can even increase our sphere of influence. If we take responsibility for a situation, it does not mean that we are the cause, or that we are to blame – rather, it means that we take responsibility for doing something about the matter. In this way, we can accept unfavourable circumstances (the reality check) but this does not mean that we approve of, or will tolerate, them. We can commit to taking whatever action is necessary to resolve the situation. This is responsibility without blame. When we begin to take responsibility, we increase our sphere of influence.

EXPANDING OUR CIRCLE OF INFLUENCE

Covey (1999) makes a distinction between proactively focused people and reactively focused people. Reactive focused people are driven by their feelings, over which they feel they have no control, and therefore have lower EQ. Proactive focused people are self-aware: they acknowledge their feelings yet remain in control of how they respond to them. They are in control of their emotional responses and therefore have higher EQ. Covey highlights this distinction in the differing attitudes towards love. He suggests that reactive people view love as a feeling. It is something that happens to them over which they have no control. They feel love but cannot 'do' love. They do not appear to generate love if it does not already exist outside of themselves. Proactive focused people, on the other hand, treat love as a verb, as something we can do.

Coaching Case Study

At one seminar where I was speaking on the concept of proactivity, a man came up and said: 'Stephen, I like what you're saying. But every situation is so different. Look at my marriage. I'm really worried. My wife and I just don't have the same feelings for each other we used to have. I guess I just don't love her anymore and she doesn't love me. What can I do?'

'The feeling isn't there anymore?' I asked.

'That's right', he reaffirmed. 'And we have three children we're really concerned about. What do you suggest?'

'Love her', I replied.

'You don't understand. The feeling of love just isn't there.'

'Then love her. If the feeling isn't there, that's good reason to love her.'

'But how do you love when you don't love?'

'My friend, love is a verb. Love-the feeling-is a fruit of love, the verb. So love her. Serve her. Sacrifice. Listen to her. Empathize. Appreciate. Affirm her. Are you willing to do that?'

(Covey, 1999)

A proactive or a reactive focus is not a fixed character trait that we cannot change. Indeed, it is entirely possible to change, and we do this by shifting our focus: by changing where we put our attention. In so doing, we begin to shift towards expanding our circle of influence. Covey suggests we consider two concentric circles. The inner circle is our area of influence, namely those things over which we exert some control. The outer circle is our circle of concern: those things which concern us, but over which we have no control, such as the threat of war or redundancy.

EXERCISE

Before reading on, take some time to make a list of all those issues that currently cause you concern. Then draw two circles, one inside the other. In the outer circle put all those issues over which you have no control whatsoever. In the inner circle put all those issues over which you do have some control. This is your circle of influence.

(I am keen to hear your experience of this exercise. If you are willing, please e-mail your feedback to ruth@dreamcoach.co.uk)

According to Covey, reactive people waste much time and energy on their circle of concern – the area over which they have no control. They spend time analysing ('Why is it like this?'), blaming ('Whose fault is it that it is like this?'), judging ('Is it right that it should be like this?'), criticising ('This is wrong, it shouldn't have to be like this, this isn't good enough'), diagnosing and prescribing ('I know what his problem is... he should get his act together').

EXERCISE

Make a note in your coaching journal every time you notice yourself analysing, blaming, judging, criticising, diagnosing and prescribing. This will develop your self-awareness. Notice how you felt at the time.

(I am keen to hear your experience of this exercise. If you are willing, please e-mail your feedback to ruth@dreamcoach.co.uk)

If you are stuck in a cycle of blaming you will become increasingly disempowered and 'victimise' yourself. You may end up in a victim role, wondering how you got there. This is the result of having a reactive focus. To make a significant shift towards proactivity, empowerment and personal responsibility, focus your time, energy and full attention on your circle of influence: on those matters in which you do exert some control. Covey (1999) observed that in adopting this approach our circle of influence actually begins to expand. Ironically, as we invest our energy only in those areas over which we have control, the area under our control begins to expand. Increasingly, more matters begin to fall into our circle of influence.

In exercising choice in how we respond to our situation, we are taking responsibility and can shift towards increasing our circle of influence. Being in a managerial role in healthcare can feel like we are sandwiched between independent professionals, over whom we have no control, on the one hand, and an inflexible bureaucracy which issues inflexible dictates on the other. We may feel powerless to intervene or to exert any influence in either direction. Yet with skill and experience we can even turn this situation into a coaching opportunity. We can expand our sphere of influence by focusing on those issues that we can change and by coaching those around us to do the same. If we are honest about our sphere of responsibility we may see that there is much that we do have control over, which we probably have not acknowledged. For example, we have a choice about our own behaviour in relation to our work colleagues.

It's the nature of reactive people to absolve themselves of responsibility. It's so much safer to say, 'I am not responsible'. If I say 'I am responsible', I might have to say, 'I am irresponsible'. It would be very hard for me to say that I have the power to choose my response and that the response I have chosen has resulted in my involvement in a negative, collusive environment, especially if for years I have absolved myself of responsibility for results in the name of someone else's weakness.

(*Covey, 1999*)

Where relationships are concerned, trying to find who is 'at fault' is a sign of emotional immaturity. In a relationship, with family and with those with whom we work, we are continually changing and growing. If the relationship is to allow for our growth then old established patterns must be challenged and changed. It is not a case of 'fault' but rather that the relationship must change to enable those within it to grow. In accepting responsibility to change our circumstances, we are not suggesting it is the fault of someone else, nor are we suggesting it is our fault either. It is not about blame but rather about healthy growth. When a houseplant outgrows the pot, the fault lies neither in the plant, nor the pot, but rather in life's own drive towards natural, healthy, growth.

When we are responsible for managing healthcare professionals, who exercise professional autonomy, coaching offers an effective management style which enables professional accountability, autonomy and responsibility to flourish.

STRESS AND PERFORMANCE

As mentioned earlier, the impact of stress on performance is such that professionals are less likely to be able to think clearly, more likely to make errors of judgement, more likely to develop stress-related illness and less likely to be flexible in their thinking. Stress narrows down our options by reducing our ability to think and create alternatives. If you want to improve your unit's sickness/absence levels and improve general performance, then take initiatives to reduce stress. Increasing control among your people by coaching them is an extremely effective method of stress reduction. The changes are tangible and permanent.

Gossip and advanced communication

Do you communicate effectively, or do you just indulge in gossip?

What is the difference? Coaching is an advanced form of communication. When we coach our colleagues we are encouraging them to become proactive. We encourage them to be creative and to generate solutions to whatever issues lie before them. So how do we distinguish between malicious gossip and genuine concern about a third party? If we are in a situation with a work colleague where we are discussing someone else, it pays to notice the focus of the conversation. We need to ask ourselves why we are discussing a third person without addressing her directly. If our attention is on her 'problems' and 'incompetencies' then we are almost certainly being drawn into gossip. It is a sign of emotional maturity to be able to resist this and to coach the person to whom we are speaking in their relationship with the third person. Specifically, we may encourage them to look at the dynamics of their relationship and encourage them to take responsibility for exploring solutions. If a colleague approaches you to discuss the 'incompetence' of another, you may ask: 'Have you coached her in this?', or 'What does she do well?'

If the person who has approached you is willing, she may appreciate your teaching her how to coach her colleague. This will improve the competencies of them both. Rarely, a colleague may need to report an unsafe condition for professional practice to you, if you are in a senior position, but more often gossip is just used as a way of releasing tension in the workplace, at someone else's expense.

You can just about measure the level of anxiety in a work system or family system by the amount of gossip. By 'gossip' I mean talk about another person, with a focus on that person's incompetence or pathology. We consolidate our relationships with one party at the expense of a third – or we attempt to dilute our anxiety by getting others in our camp. Gossip has nothing to do with intentions. Our conscious intentions may be only the best.

(Lerner, 1989)

Relationship triangles at work

An experienced coach manager learns to discern between a genuine risk to clients (potential professional incompetence), and the many other forms of gossip that colleagues will attempt to draw us into. We need to be alert to the possibility of being drawn into a relationship triangle. Lerner (1989) explains how people generally use the triangle to reduce stress in relationships, including relationships at work:

the triangle, not the dyad, is the basic unit of human emotional functioning, especially under stress.

(*Lerner, 1989*)

If you work in a stressful environment, you can be assured that there are many overlapping triangles at play in your workplace. Triangles exist to reduce anxiety and tension. The person who is drawing us into gossip may be totally unaware that she is doing so. We use relationship triangles to relieve our tension in one relationship by drawing in a third party. So, for example, if we feel irritated by our partner we may relieve our tension by calling our best friend and having a good old gossip about it. As coach managers we need to stay alert to the fact that these same dynamics are in play when our colleagues approach us to talk about their problems with their colleagues. Triangles relieve stress temporarily, but prolong the problems in relationships because the person is not being addressed directly and does not have an opportunity to change. We help the situation, not by being drawn into the triangle, but by coaching the person in how they are behaving and where their own responsibility lies in respect of the relationship.

Building a high-trust culture

Refusal to gossip also contributes to building trust within a team, ward or department. We become more trustworthy as people learn that we do not gossip, because the implication is that we will not gossip about them either. This contributes to building a 'high-trust' culture within our department, where staff trust one another and develop greater loyalty ties to one another. Covey (1999) describes a 'low-trust' culture as one that is superficial, based on what he terms a 'personality ethic'. This is where staff display superficial attitudes and behaviour – smiling to one colleague while criticising them to another. Colleagues are perceived as insincere and not genuine or authentic. In contrast, a high-trust culture is one where relationships are deep, lasting, and based on principles that Covey defines as a 'character ethic'. That is where the relationships are based on deeper principles such as respect, dignity, loyalty and caring.

Inspiring leaders and leadership

Are you a leader? You may not realise it, but you are. From the day you qualified in your chosen profession you became a role model and an inspiration for generations to follow. That is why it is important to develop your leadership abilities. As a coach manager you are one step nearer to being an inspirational leader. In the healthcare professions it is a pity that we often do not recognise great leadership. When asked who our role models are, we can often recall our colleagues who impressed us with their skill and wisdom – yet for some reason we do not consider them as leaders.

It is important that we begin to shift our perspective around this and acknowledge who the great leaders are within our respective professions.

EXERCISE

Before reading any further, ask yourself: what are the qualities of a great leader? Write them down before reading on.

(I am keen to hear your experience of this exercise. If you are willing, please e-mail your feedback to ruth@dreamcoach.co.uk)

Great leaders are those who inspire us, motivate us, empower us, have a vision and can express that vision to others with enthusiasm. You may find that many of your colleagues and, indeed, you will possess the qualities of leadership. It is no coincidence that I mention leadership qualities here, because many are congruent with the qualities of a great coach. As a coach manager you will effectively be practising your leadership skills on a daily basis. Next time someone laments the lack of leadership in the healthcare professions, remind yourself (and them) of the leadership qualities around you in your staff and colleagues. We are surrounded by untapped leadership potential and coaching is the key to releasing it. Every one of us has the ability to be a great leader of our profession if we have the courage to acknowledge and allow it.

If you are left with any doubt surrounding the benefits of adopting a coach manager style, or coaching as part of your managerial role, here is a summary of the points covered in this chapter. By adopting a coach manager style you will make a major contribution to:

- reduced stress
  - low staff turnover
  - reduced sickness/absence
  - reduced risk of litigation
- increased proactivity
- increased performance
- improved communication
- improved recruitment and retention
- improving your leadership skills
- developing leadership potential in your colleagues.

Whether you choose coaching as an aspect of your managerial role, or whether it is explicit in your job description, you stand on an exciting threshold. The coach manager has the potential to be an organisational leader and healer: a facilitator of change, healing and transformation by creating a healthy environment in the workplace. In effect, as a coach manager, you are a wizard with the power to transform people and organisations by releasing them from their mental prisons and unleashing their potential. By using your coaching skills you can inspire and motivate your people into overcoming their natural fear and resistance and boldly going to a place beyond their dreams.

Until one is committed, there is hesitancy, the chance to draw back, always ineffectiveness. Concerning all acts of initiative (and creation) there is one elementary truth, the ignorance of which kills countless ideas and splendid plans: that the moment one definitely commits oneself, then Providence moves too. All sorts of things occur to help one that would have never otherwise occurred. A whole stream of events issues from the decision, raising in one's favour all manner of unforeseen incidents and meetings and material assistance, which no man could have dreamed would come his way. I have learned a deep respect for one of Goethe's couplets:

Whatever you can do, or dream you can, begin it.
Boldness has genius, power and magic in it.

(Murray, 1951)

The cost of change is great, though not always financially. It takes great courage and sometimes personal sacrifice to change ourselves – yet, to echo Gandhi's words once more, we must indeed be the change that we wish to see in the world. Be a bold, courageous, inspirational coach manager and be amazed at the results within your own sphere of influence.

7

The evolution of a coaching culture

Never doubt that a small group of thoughtful, committed individuals can change the world. Indeed, it's the only thing that ever has.

Margaret Mead

We noted in the previous chapter that the benefits of coach management within a team or department were:

- reduced stress
  - low staff turnover
  - reduced sickness/absence
  - reduced risk of litigation
- increased proactivity
- increased performance
- improved communication
- improved recruitment and retention
- improved leadership skills.

In this chapter we will consider these benefits at organisational level. Imagine a complete paradigm shift from a bullying culture to a coaching culture. Imagine being part of a group whose norms, values and beliefs centre around nurturing one another and creating a healthy, healing environment. What might the implications be for the National Health Service as an organisation?

First, let us clarify what I mean by the term 'organisation' for our purposes here. We must remember that an organisation is its people. An organisation is a group of people who have come together to achieve a shared objective. It actually exists to serve the people within. It has been created to provide the structure, a framework and resources, within which people achieve this shared objective. It is there to provide whatever its people need, to get the job done. It is all to easy to forget this in an organisation as large as the NHS, and to feel as though it is people who serve the organisation. It is important to remember that the organisation exists to serve the needs of the people within, to enable them to achieve their shared objective in the most expedient way. So throughout this chapter when I refer to the 'organisation' I mean you and I. I use the term organisation to refer to the large, organised group of people who have come together with the shared objective of providing a healthcare service. Within this large group, each of us has a unique part to play, with unique strengths to contribute, yet we are all members of the same group, working to achieve our shared objective.

When an organisation begins to obstruct people, to stifle them in some way and to prevent them from doing their best work, it has lost sight of its original purpose. There is ongoing debate about the vision, mission and purpose of the NHS (Seedhouse, 1995). Actually the vision, mission and purpose of the people within the NHS is constantly changing because, as humanity evolves, generating new health needs, so the NHS evolves to accommodate them. The NHS could be seen as a large, growing, living organism with each staff member a healthy living cell, with its own unique purpose, within the larger organism. In this sense, the NHS has not lost sight of its vision – rather, it is evolving.

If we are to be able to stay in a flow state, functioning at our peak, within a growing, changing, evolving environment, we need to become accustomed to a climate of constant change. This has been challenging within the NHS because some of the changes have been dramatic and large-scale, resulting in stress and change fatigue. Developing a nationwide culture of coaching within the health service would serve to accommodate people's needs within a constantly changing environment. Organisation-wide coaching would enable people to make the necessary adaptations to adjust to change and remain open, flexible and adaptable. The rate of change in the NHS has been increasing exponentially, which means that the rate of change has not been constant but is actually increasing. Not only do we have more change, but we have more change more often.

In an increasingly changing environment it is no longer appropriate to cling onto a fixed knowledge base as though it were a life-raft. We need to learn how to let go of outdated knowledge and outmoded practice, and be courageous enough to embrace new ideas, technology and practice, based on the latest research. We have seen the shift towards evidence-based practice and this trend is set to continue. On a personal and organisational level we need to be at the cutting edge of our own performance, in a flow state, challenging ourselves enough to refresh our skills and develop new ones without overwhelming ourselves and becoming fatigued.

The business world is changing so rapidly that the need for expertise in specialist skills has been replaced by the need to learn and differentiate.

(Knight, 1995)

The above quote could easily apply to any business, organisation or profession as we adapt to an increasingly changing world. Evolution is how nature responds to changing environments. Organisms adapt in response to their changing environment and make the necessary adaptations to be able to survive in the new climate. If we remain with the analogy of the NHS as a living organism, we can see that this process is taking place. The NHS is constantly adapting to survive in a changing world climate. I would like us to remind ourselves, at this point, of the holistic (whole person) view of coaching. What affects one system affects the whole person. If disease affects one organ, we feel ill throughout our whole body. Similarly I would like to assert a whole-system view of the NHS. When there is dis-ease within one person, ward, department or unit, the whole organism is 'sick'. We cannot evolve the NHS by ignoring the needs of any team, group or individual within it. In the past, surgery has been attempted. There have been attempts to cut out 'diseased' units within the whole, in the hope that the whole can recover, but the underlying cause has not been treated so the disease breaks out in other parts of the body (the NHS).

By healing each cell (in this case individuals) within the organism (in this case, the NHS) then we deal with the whole organism and provide the optimum conditions for evolutionary growth. As mentioned earlier, in regard to group coaching, the focus of coaching is always the individual's growth rather than the group or organisational objectives. Through coaching, individuals grow and develop, and are enabled to more fully accomplish their role within the organisation and to contribute to the group (organisational) goals.

Let us take a few moments to look at how coaching is currently used within organisations. Lee Hecht Harrison is an international career services company which surveyed over four hundred human resource professionals to learn how coaching is used within their organisations (Lee Hecht Harrison, 2000).

The results reflect the use of coaching in organisations in the year 2000. 70% of respondents said that the reason coaching was provided was for leadership development. Over half (54%) said that coaching was offered equally to both high potential and other employees. In terms of effectiveness, 57% of respondents said coaching 'worked more often than not'. Only 5% said that coaching had been a disappointment. When asked why the use of coaching had grown over recent years, 60% of respondents commented that 'helping people improve is better than replacing them' and 54% said that 'good talent is hard to find and retain'. 79% felt that 'organizations will increasingly use coaching as part of their succession planning'. The implications for healthcare professionals are that coaching is viewed as an effective tool for leadership development and staff retention.

Slaski (2002) emphasises the importance of emotional intelligence (EQ) in the development of an organisation. If organisations are to be able to learn, grow and develop then the people that make up the organisation need particular skills and a degree of self-awareness. These are the qualities of EQ.

Organisational values set the emotional culture and climate. Empowerment and autonomy are contingent on emotional independence, self-awareness and self-acceptance. The success of open communications, team-working, forums and circles are dependent upon the quality of emotional relationships between individuals.

(Slaski, 2002)

BLAME

A 'blame' culture is indicative of low EQ in an organisation. When we are quick to blame we are being judgemental, making assumptions, jumping to conclusions and not accepting personal responsibility. Our thinking patterns are fixed and narrow. This is also symptomatic of a high stress environment in which people are emotionally aroused. Goleman (1996) describes a direct relationship between our level of emotional arousal and our ability to consider alternative points of view. Paradoxically, when we are emotionally aroused, our emotional brain has been stimulated by the smallest amount of information, yet the more aroused we become, the more convinced we are that we are 'right' beyond doubt. This increasing sense of self-righteousness proportional to our emotional arousal is illustrated beautifully in the following poem by Valerie Cox:

The Cookie Thief

The woman was waiting at the airport one night,
With several long hours before her flight,
She hunted for a book in the airport shop,
Bought a bag of cookies and found a place to drop.

She was engrossed in her book, but happened to see
That the man beside her, as bold as he could be,
Grabbed a cookie or two from the bag between,
Which she tried to ignore, to avoid a scene.

She read, munched cookies and watched the clock,
As the gutsy 'cookie thief' diminished her stock.
She was getting more irritated as the minutes ticked by,
Thinking, 'If I wasn't so nice, I'd blacken his eye!'

With each cookie she took, he took one, too.
When only one was left, she wondered what he'd do.
With a smile on his face and a nervous laugh,
He took the last cookie and broke it in half.

He offered her half, as he ate the other.
She snatched it from him and thought, 'Oh brother,
This guy has some nerve, and he's also rude.
Why he didn't even show any gratitude!'

She had never known when she had been so galled,
And sighed with relief when her flight was called.
She gathered her belongings and headed for the gate,
Refusing to look back at the 'thieving ingrate'.

She boarded the plane and sank in her seat,
Then sought her book, which was almost complete.
As she reached in her baggage, she gasped with surprise.
There was her bag of cookies in front of her eyes!

'If mine are here', she moaned with despair,
'Then the others were his and he tried to share!'
Too late to apologise, she realised with grief
That she was the rude one, the ingrate, the thief!

(From A Third Serving of Chicken Soup for the Soul (1996) by Jack Canfield and Mark Victor Hansen. Published with kind permission of Vermillion publishers.)

As we calm down we become cognisant again. Our emotional brain releases its grip on the cortex and we become able to think clearly again. We become aware of, and able to process, other factors and may realise that we were not so 'right' after all. If the character in the poem had not been so irate, she may have had the presence of mind to check in her bag for her own cookies in the first instance! Our emotions can actually blind us to the reality of a situation. Having higher EQ means we possess an ability to control our responses to emotions so that we are less susceptible to such 'emotional hijackings' and are able to think clearly, even under duress.

When a larger percentage of individuals within the organisation possess higher EQ, this raises the EQ of the organisation. People are less likely to blame others and more likely to accept the reality of the situation and take personal responsibility for creating a solution.

In order to evolve, and to avoid extinction, our NHS organism needs to learn to adapt to its changing environment. In order to survive, the organisation needs to develop an awareness of the external conditions which affect its existence, and to discover what adaptations it needs to make to ensure its survival and continued evolution.

THE LEARNING ORGANISATION

There are two basic schools of thought about how organisations evolve (Santos, 2002). One school suggests that the organisation has little or no control and is totally at the mercy of external forces. If the market no longer requires the products or services that the organisation provides, it will simply disappear, to be replaced with a new organisation.

The second school of thought suggests that organisations can adapt in response to external influences and can therefore change and survive. To be successful the organisation needs to continually review the external conditions that affect it, and it needs to learn how to respond. In order to survive and evolve, our NHS organism needs to learn how to learn. It needs to become a learning organisation.

Slaski (2002) suggests that a learning organisation has the following characteristics:

- *Strong customer focus*
- *Empowerment and autonomy*
- *Entrepreneurship*
- *Team-working*
- *Creativity*
- *Culture of trust and respect*
- *People development*
- *Forums and circles*
- *Continuous improvement*
- *Change management*
- *Communicating a vision*
- *Clear values and objectives*
- *Participation and involvement*
- *Open communications and networking*
- *Shared learning and knowledge.*

(Slaski, 2002)

It would seem like a quantum leap to shift from an organisation with a closed, rigid, low-trust, bullying culture which stifles creativity and communication, to an open learning organisation defined by its openness, clear communication, flexibility, high trust and respect, which enables creativity. Yet this is precisely the leap that the NHS has to make if it is to succeed in recruiting the people it needs to provide the healthcare services of the future. The NHS needs to become a healthy organism in which its cells (people) are nurtured and thrive, rather than wither and die. Through the process of affirmative inquiry, acknowledgement and structure, coaching not only provides the nutrient which our organism needs to survive but provides a method of administration.

Speaking to the Royal College of Midwives' annual conference in Bournemouth in 2002, President Lorna Muirhead DBE spoke of this lack of 'nourishment' in her presidential address:

I felt as though I had given everything I had to the NHS and to midwifery, and I felt as though I was a tree whose roots for too long had had little or no fertilisation.

(Muirhead, 2002)

Will our NHS organism adapt and evolve, or will it become extinct? Recruitment of essential personnel is going to be a key factor in our organism's fight for survival. Recruitment is how our organism 'grows' healthy new cells. The maternity services provide an excellent illustration of the challenges faced by our NHS organism. Dimond (2002) describes some issues which influenced the recruitment of midwives during 2002. Of 141 maternity units in the UK 88% were experiencing some level of staffing shortage compared to 76% in 2001. The recruitment problem is getting worse. The largest group of midwives leaving the NHS gave 'dissatisfaction with midwifery' as the reason. Among the main causes of this dissatisfaction were:

- a lack of support from managers
- unwillingness to practise the type of midwifery that the NHS demands, and
- dissatisfaction with the requirement to rotate through shifts and departments.

In a coaching culture, each of these factors are addressed. Coaching itself, with its emphasis on affirmative inquiry, provides essential support to and from managers throughout the organisational structure. The autonomy and empowerment provided through coaching affords practitioners autonomy and flexibility. They are not 'required' to practise any form of midwifery other than that which they feel is most appropriate. They have greater autonomy in clinical decision-making. Finally, the focus on strengths means that each individual is doing what they do best most of the time. They would not be required to 'rotate' into unfamiliar areas which would diminish their performance. This may mean a radical re-think of how midwifery is practised in the UK. It may mean considering doing things differently than we have ever done before, or revisiting methods that worked in a previous time to review them from our new perspective. This is the essence of evolution – doing whatever we need to do in order to survive.

Coaching offers a method for managers and peers to provide the essential acknowledgement that is so lacking in the present NHS. Speaking of midwives in particular, Dame Lorna Muirhead commented:

They have given everything they have. They have adapted the way they practise, changed their work patterns, organised their children, cleaned their homes, looked after aging parents, kept professionally up to date, maintained their PREP folder, or done a degree. They have done everything the profession and the service has asked of them, and it is still not enough, because the sheer volume of work is oppressive.

(Muirhead, 2002)

This suggests that the NHS, as an organisation, is acting counter-productively in restricting the performance of its people. To succeed in its aim of providing a maternity service, the role of the organisation is to create an environment conducive to recruitment which will attract high-calibre midwives, then create structures which nurture and enable them to perform to the best of their ability. In a climate in which you can give everything you have and yet feel that it is not enough, and will never be enough, acknowledgement of your dedication, commitment and effort is especially important. It is essential. Effective coaching, leading to a higher EQ throughout the NHS, may not only be desirable but may be essential for the survival of the NHS.

Reviewing the characteristics [of a learning organisation] it is hard to see how any of these can be achieved without some consideration as to the role of emotions. Teamwork, trust, sharing, creativity, autonomy, communicating, are all characteristics heavy in emotional content... The success of open communications, team-working, forums and circles are dependent upon the quality of emotional relationships between individuals.

(Slaski, 2002)

A COACHING CULTURE IN THE NHS

As mentioned earlier in this book, culture is defined by sociologists as:

The values, beliefs, customs, rules and regulations of a group or society

(Haralambos, 1986)

Every group of people, ranging from a family to a large organisation such as the NHS, has its own codes of behaviour, expressed as 'the way we do things around here'. These rules, which can be formal or informal, explicit or implied, are enforced by the use of sanctions. We conform to the group norms or sanctions are applied. With formal rules, which are set out and made explicit (such as your organisation's policy), the sanctions are usually equally formal and explicit (such as your organisation's disciplinary procedure). If we break the group rules, there will be consequences.

With informal 'rules', which may be subtle expected standards of behaviour that are implicit, this becomes more complex. The group may not expressly tell us how to behave, but we feel the consequences when we mis-read the signs and breach the 'rules'. Look at your own family as an example. You know what standards of behaviour are expected within your family and how these may differ from behaviour in other families. You also know from experience the consequences of stepping out of line. Sanctions are applied.

In the healthcare professions, new members learn the codes of behaviour necessary to be accepted to the group. They must quickly learn the group 'norms' if they wish to be accepted into the group. A failure to do this results in exclusion from the group and/or applied sanctions. If this sounds primordial and uncivilised – it is. Our emotional brains are ancient and primitive. Remember:

Twenty-first century man is really a 'space-age man with a stone age constitution'

(Slaski, 2002)

In the NHS, our immature attempts to sanction group members manifest as the bullying culture (Hadikin and O'Driscoll, 2000). In order to understand where we are going with NHS culture it is first important to understand where we have been, how we got here, and where we are now. In effect we will take a 'reality check' of our organisational culture at this point.

A combination of historical and sociological factors contributed to the development of the present culture within the NHS. Two of the informal, unspoken, implicit 'rules' which still apply within NHS culture are:

- obey without question, and
- always put others first (self-sacrifice).

Let us take a moment here to explore the origins of these beliefs.

Obey without question

In the army, the culture is one of not questioning officers of senior rank. This is illustrated in the axiom: 'When I say jump, you jump.' With early hospitals historically arising from army field hospitals, it became an unspoken 'rule' that doctors and nurses (who were often considered senior in terms of rank and/or social class) knew best, and their authority was not to be questioned, least of all by their patients (Hadikin and O'Driscoll, 2000).

Self-sacrifice

The influence of the Church on early nineteenth and twentieth century nursing sisters resulted in a strong emphasis on obedience, poverty and selflessness. This is still echoed today when people express the fear that 'if you pay nurses too much you might attract people who are only in it for the money' (Hadikin and O'Driscoll, 2000).

The emphasis on sacrificing the self, while demanding unquestioning obedience to authority, placed early healthcare practitioners in an extremely disempowering position and still does to a greater or lesser degree. This contributes to the 'high pressure – low control' condition which is so detrimental to health. It contributes to a feeling of disempowerment and perpetuates the erroneous belief that there is nothing we can do to change our circumstances. It takes all control out of the hands of the individual and places control in the hands of their superiors and even external circumstances such as the workload.

Shifting perspective

To integrate a coaching culture within the NHS, some of the existing norms, beliefs and values must first be challenged. We must first work on ourselves and on challenging our own beliefs. Then we must have the courage to challenge existing practice, not only in a clinical sense, but in a cultural sense too. We must have the courage to challenge existing routines.

I spoke with a client last night who told me about a midwife who was being persecuted by a family in her neighbourhood. The family perceived she had wronged them in some way. She was understandably distressed, since her children were being targeted at school by this family and, in her words, 'it is becoming a nightmare'. My client was convinced that there was nothing this midwife could do, and the matter was beyond her control, because she was the victim in this case.

This offers an interesting example for us to illustrate the concept of control. Certainly, the midwife has been the target of a personal attack. Whether she is a victim or not is her choice. It depends on how she reacts or responds to her situation. It is her choice whether to continue to tolerate this family's behaviour, or whether she does something about it. If she chooses to suffer, to tolerate, to stay in a situation that could harm her and her family, to tolerate damage and harm, then she will certainly become a victim. If she succumbs to fear she will become a victim. If she takes action to address the issue (whatever the nature of the action) then she is no longer a victim.

Coaching can bring a change in perspective to healthcare provision as a whole, empowering professionals by gradually replacing the passive 'there is nothing we can do' belief with one of 'there is always something we can do'.

EXERCISE

How aware are you of the norms, values and beliefs in your working environment? Not the rhetoric. Not what is supposed to happen according to the textbooks. Not what you think should happen in an ideal world, but what actually does happen. Here and now. What is the reality in your workplace? How do you usually do things?

Read the following value statements and note which ones most closely resemble the attitudes in your workplace. You can choose as many as you like and/or create your own.

'We get through the work as quick as possible, then we can have a cup of tea.'

'We like to share the work out equally.'

'We are proud of our client-centred approach.'

'We pay lip service to a patient-centred approach but everyone knows we're really just getting by as best we can.'

'We support and nurture each other.'

'If you can't stand the heat, you shouldn't be in the kitchen.'

'It's every man for himself around here.'

'We're proud that all our clients are seen within five minutes of their appointment time.'

'We are proud that we spend time with our clients and they appreciate it. So what if they have to wait a bit longer to be seen, they really don't mind.'

Create five or six statements, similar to those above, that would accurately reflect the values and beliefs of your place of work. Take into account the whole team or ward, not just your opinion. That is your group culture.

(I am keen to hear your experience of this exercise. If you are willing, please e-mail your feedback to ruth@dreamcoach.co.uk)

In returning to our analogy of an organism, the culture can be viewed as the invisible threads that hold the organism together. The spirit or soul of the organisation. Irrespective of whether the organisational objectives are met, the organisation will hold together, provided the culture is one which nurtures the people within. If the culture is one which is negative, it can destroy the organisation from within.

Santos (2002) emphasises the importance of timing. It is still possible for an organisation to become extinct if the necessary action is taken too late. To ensure an organisation's survival, any initiatives to adapt and respond to the environment must be appropriate and timely.

This chapter has outlined some of the ways that coaching can be used as a valuable tool to enable the NHS to respond to external circumstances and ensure its continued survival as an organisation. The following chapter looks at some of the national and global health trends to which the NHS may need to respond in the future, if indeed it is to survive and evolve, and the part coaching can play in such a transformation.

8

Future visions: the future role of coaching in healthcare

By learning to better love and care for ourselves as well as each other, we get closer to that which is greater than any one of us. When we serve and foster one soul, we serve the whole world.

Lama Surya Das

As mentioned in the preceding chapter, culture represents the norms, values and beliefs of a group. One of the biggest trends which influences the way humanity evolves is group size. Increasingly, we live in larger and larger groups, and we continually develop new skills which enable us to do this. Historically, we evolved from small groups of hunter-gatherers, through to agricultural peoples living in small villages, to large civilisations living in cities. In cultural terms, we shifted from identifying ourselves as a family, to identifying ourselves as a tribe and eventually as a nation. At this point in time, the beginning of the twenty-first century, we can see certain trends. We can see that we are developing into a global culture. We will need to learn a new skill set that enables us to transcend nationalism and develop a global identity. How does this relate to coaching? Coaching is an advanced mode of communication and as such, may well be facilitating our evolution. The future is not predictable and for ease of writing (and reading) this chapter is based on the assumption that current observable trends are set to continue.

It has been noted that humans use language to enable them to form strong kinship bonds and loyalty ties, much as other primates might use grooming behaviour (Dunbar, 1996). Primates use grooming and physical touch to bond with one another. As early humans evolved from small intimate family groups to larger tribes, we needed to develop a different method of bonding with each other. Dunbar (1996) explains how language evolved in response to our evolutionary need for a way to bond with large numbers of people with whom we may never have physical contact. Essentially, we 'groom' each other with our language and this enables us to bond with one another and to form loyalty ties. We use the term 'networking' to describe the process of setting up and maintaining a support network for ourselves. We also noted earlier in this book that some people are more effective networkers than others, and therefore have a stronger support network. These people are developing new skills which enable them to connect with large numbers of people. They are developing emotional intelligence (EQ).

As we make the evolutionary transition toward a global culture, our language, and our whole way of connecting with one another, must evolve accordingly to enable us to bond with greater numbers of people than ever before. EQ may be the next phase of our own evolution. It certainly plays a key role in our ability to bond with people. Large numbers of people, indeed the whole of humanity, may be evolving towards higher EQ. At this point in time, coaching has emerged as a tool which facilitates this process. In future, coaching may become a way of life. We may each have our favourite personal coach whom we see regularly, much like we would hire a hairdresser today, or it may be that the process of coaching itself becomes a normal part of our communication skills. At such time when the whole population possesses sufficient EQ, and effective coaching skills, we may facilitate one another's development without hiring an outside 'expert'. We may not use the term coaching but, in one form or another, this advanced skill set that leads to emotional intelligence will become a normal part of our lives by the end of the twenty-first century.

As the trend towards a global community progresses, we will increasingly identify with a global culture. We will move increasingly towards a set of norms, values and beliefs that will be agreed upon globally. There will always be sub-cultures as smaller groups exist within the larger group, and our national identity may indeed become an aspect of sub-culture, but our mainstream culture will increasingly be global in origin. If we are to move towards a set of values, beliefs and behaviour 'norms' that are generally agreed upon at global level there must be significant paradigm shifts from our current belief systems. There is some evidence that this is happening. There seems to be a convergence, or homogenisation, of beliefs and philosophies. Certainly there appears to be a merging of eastern and western belief which is currently informing our approach to healthcare. The future may see a continuing paradigm shift in mainstream culture, away from curing, towards healing. We are already witnessing the move away from the medical 'expert' and a trend towards self-healing, personal responsibility, alternative and complementary therapies. Ideas, beliefs, values and practices in relation to health may spread remarkably quickly from one part of the world to another.

There may be a global paradigm shift in medicine away from 'systems' thinking and toward holistic medicine. This philosophy may also affect our view of organisations. We may increasingly view our bodies, our organisations and our world holistically: as one huge, interconnected, living organism.

The stories, myths, beliefs, values and norms that form our culture are the threads that bind us together as a group. Once we begin to challenge these, and outmoded ideas begin to disintegrate, the world becomes an unpredictable place. Once our traditional bonds are broken our foundations become shaky. Fear and anxiety rise due to the uncertainty of the future. In order to smooth the transition to a new culture, we need to consciously create and embrace our new values, beliefs and norms. This is nothing new. We have evolved this way over many centuries. As each generation challenges the beliefs of previous generations, we make significant paradigm shifts that influence our culture. What is remarkable is the speed of such change in the present day. Global communications, especially television, film, and the internet, play a huge part in creating this sense of global community. Values, beliefs and behaviour norms, the very basis of culture, are generated and perpetuated through the media.

A new term has arisen which describes this concept of consciously, and deliberately, creating our own culture: the Cultural Creative. Humans have become a species of Cultural Creatives. We create our own culture, and set up the structures, rules and routines, which eventually guide our own evolution. We are not merely aware of a process which is beyond our control: we are controlling this process. Perhaps for the first time in history we are conscious of the fact that we are influencing our own evolution. Our choices matter. This contributes to an increased sense of personal responsibility and power.

The observable trends which I have outlined here are:

- a trend towards holism
- increased personal responsibility
- an increasing awareness that our choices affect our evolution
- an increased feeling of connectedness with other peoples worldwide
- an increase in global communication.

These are the drivers which are guiding our evolution. Our desire to connect with others on a global level, and our desire to understand them, are the factors which are driving our need to develop greater emotional intelligence. These are the external conditions which, in turn, are driving the evolution of the health service as an organisation.

Let us take a moment to examine the implications of these trends on a personal, professional and organisational level. How will these changes affect us?

On a personal level, we will see wider choices for ourselves in healthcare. We may increasingly use alternative and complementary therapies ourselves. We may develop an increased awareness of our own health and accept more responsibility for maintaining our health and preventing ill-health. We may have fewer occasions of illness and, when we do become ill, we may be less likely to consult an expert and more likely to know what to do for ourselves. An example might be that we no longer see our family doctor for many complaints, and we may prefer to use naturopathic remedies instead.

We may become more open-minded and willing to consider new and different approaches to our health. Our developing EQ and ability to connect globally might mean we adopt health practices from other cultures and share health practices with other nations and cultures. We may integrate many health practices. If we have positive experience of holistic medicine ourselves, we may readily integrate complementary therapies into our practice. Indeed some 'complementary' techniques may no longer be viewed as 'complementary' to traditional medicine but may become part of our traditional approach to health.

On a personal level we may:

- increase our use of holistic medicine
- increase our focus on self-care
- have increased knowledge of our personal health and wellbeing

- have increased willingness to try new and different ideas
- have higher EQ
- have balance between work and personal life
- have more focus on integrating personal values into our work
- have an increased desire for satisfying and fulfilling occupations.

The concept of 'complementary' medicine itself reflects our current culture. If a health initiative or practice is widely adopted in another culture (Chinese medicine, for example) it is regarded as complementary to our own. With increasing global communication, shared knowledge and evidence-based practice, the emphasis will increasingly be on whatever method is most effective, irrespective of its country of origin. Many so-called complementary therapies may well be researched and in future adopted as 'best practice'.

Many unusual health practices are currently being examined for effectiveness. There is a resurgence of interest in distance healing at the time of writing. What had traditionally been viewed with some scepticism, and largely dismissed as 'faith healing', has been given some credibility – paradoxically, by the latest ideas in physics. Scientists are, unintentionally, lending credibility to the idea that it is possible to heal from a distance. Contemporary physicists suggest that there is no such thing as empty space. Between you and I, there is no space. The very air we breathe is full of minute particles and energy, some of which pass through our bodies as they travel through the universe. Respected scientists such as Dr David Bohm (1980) suggest that 'everything in the universe affects everything else because they are all part of the same unbroken whole'. This has led to a new surge of interest in discovering whether distance healing could work, and how, rather than the previously dismissive attitude. It suggests that something more is involved rather than just 'auto-suggestion' or hypnosis.

The idea is that there could be a transference of 'healthy' energy somehow from the healthy individual, or healer, to the sick individual. This is very far-fetched and sounds like science fiction, yet there is ongoing research examining this type of 'energy' healing (Schlitz and Braud, 1997; Sicher et al, 1998; Harris et al, 1999). The healthcare practitioner of the future may become a healer.

What would be the implications for healthcare practice? With clients increasingly responsible for themselves, and greater interest in complementary health and even healers, the traditional role of healthcare practitioners could diminish. People may suffer fewer episodes of illness and when they do they may resort to gentler healing approaches rather than invasive surgery or pharmaceuticals. There may be smaller core units with a few core staff and more healthcare professionals may be self-employed in private practice or associated with the NHS. This implies a period of change, learning and transformation for people already in and entering the healthcare professions. Coaching offers an effective tool to facilitate this transition and a coaching culture creates the optimum learning environment for this transformation to take place. Indeed, the role of the healthcare practitioner may well be one of coach, advisor and consultant as the focus shifts from 'doing for' our clients to enabling them to 'do for' themselves.

Factors affecting healthcare professionals in future may be:

- increased personal responsibility for health
- changing role of healthcare professional to that of coach/consultant
- increased awareness of health
- fewer episodes of illness
- increase in self-employed healthcare professionals
- need to develop business/leadership skills
- increased EQ
- increased need to learn.

Some of these trends are apparent already. As television, the internet and mass communication spreads beliefs and ideas about health on a global level, people will increasingly become aware of 'what works' in terms of healthy living. The current boom in health-related industries, from health foods to gymnasiums, is set to continue as increasingly large numbers of people become conscious of how to maintain good health. This will, in the long term, reduce the demands on the NHS and the need for healthcare professionals as we know them today. The role of the healer, which has until now been marginalised, may well take centre stage. We can see this trend already with healers collaborating with doctors to provide healing services in GP surgeries (see doctor-healer network in the Resources section of this book). This implies an evolving role for a healthcare practitioner who is, in effect, a healer, coach and health advisor (though we may not use those terms).

Now let us consider the implications for the evolving organisation. As mentioned earlier, changes in the mainstream culture become a driver of organisational change or evolution. The organisation must adapt to external conditions if it is to survive. As mentioned in the previous chapter, the organisation must become a learning organisation. This means the organisation of the future needs:

- more collaborative working
- increased openness
- more teamworking
- better communication
- higher EQ
- to capitalise on creativity
- to learn how to learn
- to be strengths-based
- to develop a coaching culture.

In the process of becoming a learning organisation, our NHS 'organism' will need to learn how to learn, in order to remain responsive to the ever-changing external conditions. This means fully utilising the people within the organisation by enabling them to work in the flow, use their strengths on a daily basis and develop their creativity. Essentially, employees will need to become 'intrapreneurs'.

THE 'INTRAPRENEUR'

Entrepreneurs are basically ideas people. A true entrepreneur is as much 'in love' with ideas themselves as she is with making profit. Entrepreneurs are creative people who generate ideas and innovate. Typically they will either sell a business, or put a manager in place, to enable them to move on to their next idea. We have such people working within large organisations such as the NHS. We have wonderfully creative 'ideas people', but we do not offer an outlet for their creativity. The concept of the 'intrapreneur' involves incorporating a philosophy and a framework which enables the untapped creativity of people working within organisations to be released.

Through the choices we make, we are effectively steering our own evolution. We are controlling our own evolution by controlling our environment. It is our choice whether we overcome our barriers to communication, heal our negative organisational cultures and raise our EQ. Once we have achieved this, our lives become easier. We no longer struggle over difficult relationships at work. It becomes easier to interact with difficult people and, once the organisation raises its overall EQ, there are fewer 'difficult' people around. This releases our creative energy so that we are free to become 'intrapreneurs' (creative innovators) within our organisation. It is our choice whether we learn the necessary skills to become self-employed and use our creativity to develop initiatives which are responsive to the health demands of the future. The choices we make now affect how our future will look.

ENVISIONING A HEALTHY NHS

Take a moment now to consider your vision for our future. What do you envision for your grandchildren, and great-grandchildren, in terms of healthy living?

As you may have gathered, my vision is one where everyone has access to accurate information about how to stay in good health and avoid sickness. My vision is one where healing is a gentle art, practised without adding harm to the 'sick'. My vision is one where healing is initiated from within, through living in a healthy, nurturing environment. Coaching plays a pivotal role in my vision for our future. Within an organisation that is based on a coaching culture, we are free to explore and create the best practices to generate health.

Coaching reconnects us with who we really are. It enables us to define our sense of self. Coaching has the potential to reconnect us with our personal values, our beliefs, our spirituality and our vision. I envision the NHS of the future as an organisation which exists to promote and maintain good health by offering advice, information and coaching in addition to providing emergency care and core services. In my vision, there may be many self-employed practitioners who work with the NHS, contributing to an environment of healing and growth. The NHS of the future may be a knowledge and resource base: informing and coaching us toward total physical, mental, emotional and spiritual health. In my vision, the NHS leads by example: the NHS would create a healthy nurturing environment in which all its employees and associates experience physical, mental, emotional and spiritual wellbeing themselves and are able to convey this to their clients. The NHS would project a healthy 'energy' which 'infects' all who come into contact with it. This wouldn't happen by 'magic' – this would happen through an effective coaching culture. Through a coaching culture we would first learn how to nurture ourselves, and each other, and then we could enable our clients to do the same. Just imagine!

The future of organizational development belongs to methods that affirm, compel, and accelerate anticipatory learning involving larger and larger levels of collectivity. The new methods will be distinguished by the art and science of asking powerful, positive questions.

(Cooperrider and Pratt, 1987)

At this current point in time we are using the term coaching to describe this art and science of asking questions that empower, motivate and facilitate our growth and development. So now, at the end of this book, what does the term coaching mean to you?

- Coaching can be a skill set.
- It can be a management style.
- It can be a communication style.
- It can be a philosophy.
- It can be a process of affirmative appreciative, inquiry which, as Hubbard (1998) suggests, 'seeks out the best of "what is" in order to ignite the collective imagination of "what might be"'.

Coaching can be all of this, and it can be the light which illuminates our vision.

In coaching, we begin with our vision. Then we take our reality check. Then we ask ourselves: what do we need in order to get from where we are now, to where we want to be? Effective coaching, that leads to physical, mental, emotional and spiritual growth, is what we need now to move forward to our vision.

References

Bohm D 1980 Wholeness and the implicate order. Routledge & Kegan Paul, London

Bowen M 1978 Family therapy in clinical practice. Jason Aronson, New York

Brendgen J 2002 Overcoming low self esteem: a cognitive behavioural approach. Stress News 14 (3): 7- 11

Buckingham M, Clifton D O 2002. Now discover your strengths: how to develop your talents and those of the people you manage. Simon & Schuster, London

Carson R D 1990 Taming your gremlin: a guide to enjoying yourself. Harper Perennial, New York

Coaches Training Institute 2002 The co-active coaching model. http://www.thecoaches.com/registration/coaching.html (accessed 4 Oct 2002)

CoachU Inc 1999 Coach training program (CTP). Modules 1-36. CoachU Inc, Salina, KS

Covey S R 1999 The 7 habits of highly effective people. Simon & Schuster, London

Cox V 1996 The cookie thief. In: Hansen J, Canfield V, Hansen MV (eds) A Third Helping of Chicken Soup for the Soul. Health Communications Inc, Deerfield Beach, FL

Davies J B 1992 The myth of addiction: an application of the psychological theory of attribution to illicit drug use. Routledge, London

Department of the Environment 1995 Deprivation index: a review of approaches and matrix of results. HMSO, London

Dimond B 2002 Staffing, stress, bullying and the midwife. British Journal of Midwifery 10 (11): 710-713

Douglas M 2002 Unpublished ongoing research. http://www.clinicaltrials.gov/ct/gui/show/NCT00012896;jsessionid=70EBBE558DCF8C91262B67C61DCB39FF?order=1 (accessed 28 Dec 2002)

Dunbar R 1996 Grooming, gossip and the evolution of language. Faber & Faber, London

Festinger L 1957 A theory of cognitive dissonance. Harper, New York

Festinger L, Carlsmith J M 1959 Cognitive consequences of forced compliance. Journal of Abnormal and Social Psychology 58: 203-210

Frankl V E 1997 Man's search for meaning, revised and updated edition [originally published 1946] Washington Square Press, New York

Gallwey W T 1997 The inner game of tennis. Random House, New York

Goleman D 1996 Emotional intelligence: why it can matter more than IQ. Bloomsbury, London

Hadikin R 2002 10 steps to personal power. Nursing Times 98 (32): 26-27

Hadikin R, O'Driscoll M 2000 The bullying culture. Books For Midwives, Oxford

Haralambos M 1986 Sociology: a new approach. Causeway Press, Ormskirk

Harris W S, Gowda M, Kolb J W et al 1999 A randomized, controlled trial of the effects of remote, intercessory prayer on outcomes in patients admitted to the coronary care unit. Archives of Internal Medicine 160 (12): 1878

Heider F 1958 The psychology of interpersonal relationships. Lawrence Erlbaum, Mahweh, NJ

Herman J L 1992 Trauma and recovery. Basic Books, New York

Hubbard B M 1998 Conscious evolution: awakening the power of our social potential. New World Library, Novato, CA

International Coach Federation 2002 The nature and scope of coaching. http://www.coachfederation.org/aboutcoaching/nature.htm and http://www.coachfederation.org/credentialing/en/core.htm (accessed 16 Jul 2002)

Illich I 1971 Deschooling society. Harper & Row, New York

Katie B 2002 Loving what is: four questions that can change your life. Rider, London

Kelley R, Caplan J 1993 How Bell Labs creates star performers. Harvard Business Review July-Aug 1993. Cited in: Goleman D 1996 Emotional intelligence: why it can matter more than IQ. Bloomsbury, London

Knight S 1995 NLP at work. Nicholas Brearley Publishing, London

Landsberg M 1996 The tao of coaching: boost your effectiveness at work by inspiring and developing those around you. Harper Collins Business, London

Lee Hecht Harrison 2000 How is coaching used in your organisation? http://www.lhh.com/us/rsrchinfo/studies/srvyresults.html (accessed 21 Jun 2002)

Lerner H 1989 The dance of intimacy. Harper and Row, New York

Lerner H 1990 The dance of anger: a guide to changing the pattern of intimate relationships. Thorsons, London

Maslow A H 1982 Toward a psychology of being, 2nd edn. Nostrand Reinhold, New York

Muirhead L 2002 Honouring midwifery - a pause for thought. RCM Midwives Journal 5 (7): 224-227

Murray W H 1951 The Scottish Himalayan expedition. J M Dent and Sons Ltd, New York

Nagy J 2001 [unpublished] Speaking on 'financial independence' teleclass 19 Jul 2001. CoachU Inc, Salina, KS

Pearsall J, Trumble B (eds) 1996 The Oxford English reference dictionary, 2nd edn. Oxford University Press, Oxford

Peck M S 1990 The road less travelled: the new psychology of love, traditional values and spiritual growth. Arrow Books, London

Rogers C 1961 On becoming a person: a therapist's view of psychotherapy. Constable, London

Salovey P, Mayer J D 1990 Emotional intelligence. Imagination, Cognition and Personality 9 (3): 185-211

Santos A M 2002 The phenomenon of organizational evolution: a model for analysis. Leadership & Organisational Development Journal 23 (4): 215-227

Schlitz M, Braud W 1997 Distant intentionality and healing: assessing the evidence. Alternative Therapies in Health and Medicine 3 (6): 62-73

Seedhouse D 1995 Fortress NHS: a philosophical review of the national health service. Wiley, Chichester

Sicher F, Targ E, Moore D 2nd, Smith H S 1998 A randomized double-blind study of the effect of distant healing in a population with advanced AIDS. Report of a small scale study. Western Journal of Medicine 169 (6): 356-363

Smith J, Palmer S 2000 Stress management coach validation consultation process. Stress News 12 (4): 7

Slaski M, Cartwright S 2002 Health, performance and emotional intelligence: an exploratory study of retail managers. Stress and Health 18: 63-68

Slaski M 2002 Emotional intelligence: is it a concept that can be used in stress management? Stress News 14 (3): 13-15

Vale M J et al 2002 Coaching patients with coronary heart disease to achieve the target cholesterol: a method to bridge the gap between evidence-based medicine and the 'real world'. Journal of Clinical Epidemiology 55: 245-252

Whittemore R, Chase S A, Mandle C L et al 2001 The integrity and efficacy of a nurse-coaching intervention in type 2 diabetes. The Diabetes Educator 27: 887-898

Whitmore J 1996 Coaching for performance. Nicholas Brearley Publishing, London

Whitworth L, Kimsey-House H, Sandahl P 1998 Co-active coaching: new skills for coaching people toward success in work and life. Davies-Black Publishing, Palo Alta, CA

Further reading

Benner P 1984 From novice to expert: excellence and power in clinical nursing practice. Addison-Wesley, Menlo Park, CA, p 77-94

Buckingham M, Clifton D O 2002 Now discover your strengths: how to develop your talents and those of the people you manage. Simon & Schuster, London

Fortgang L B 1998 Take yourself to the top. Thorsons, London

Goleman D 1996 Emotional intelligence: why it can matter more than IQ. Bloomsbury, London

Hadikin R 2002 10 steps to personal power. Nursing Times 98 (32): 26-27

Hadikin R, O'Driscoll M 2000 The bullying culture. Books For Midwives, Oxford

Leonard T J 1998 The portable coach. Scribner, New York

Lerner H 1990 The dance of anger: a guide to changing the pattern of intimate relationships. Thorsons, London

Lewis F M, Zahlis E H 1997 The nurse as coach: A conceptual framework for clinical practice. Oncology Nursing Forum 24: 1695-1702

Maslow A H 1982 Toward a psychology of being, 2nd edn. Nostrand Reinhold, New York

Parker-Loewen P L, Lytton H 1987 Effects of short-term interaction coaching with mothers of preterm infants. Infant Mental Health Journal 8: 277-287

Samarel N, Fawcett J 1992 Enhancing adaptation to breast cancer: the addition of coaching to support groups. Oncology Nursing Forum 19: 591-596

Samarel N, Fawcett J, Tulman L 1993 The effects of coaching in breast cancer support groups: a pilot study. Oncology Nursing Forum 20: 795-798

Samarel N, Fawcett J, Tulman L 1997 Effect of support groups with coaching on adaptation to early stage breast cancer. Research in Nursing and Health 20: 15-26

Vale M J et al 2002 Coaching patients with coronary heart disease to achieve the target cholesterol: a method to bridge the gap between evidence-based medicine and the 'real world'. Journal of Clinical Epidemiology 55: 245-252

Whitmore J 1996 Coaching for performance. Nicholas Brealey Publishing, London

Whitworth L, Kimsey-House H, Sandahl P 1998 Co-active coaching: new skills for coaching people toward success in work and life. Davies-Black Publishing, Palo Alta, CA

Wilkie DJ, Williams AR, Grevstad P et al 1995 Coaching persons with lung cancer to report sensory pain. Cancer Nursing 18: 7-15

Resources/websites

Professional associations for coaches

Association For Coaching
Tel: +44 (0)207 259 2798 (UK)
enquiries@associationforcoaching.com
www.associationforcoaching.com

The European Mentoring and Coaching Council
www.emccouncil.org

International Coach Federation
Tel: 1-888-423-3131 (USA)
icfoffice@coachfederation.org
www.coachfederation.org

Coach training organisations

CoachU
www.coachueurope.com

International Coach Academy
www.icoachacademy.co.uk and www.icoachacademy.com

Life Coach School International
www.lifecoachschoolinternational.co.uk

The Coaching Academy UK Ltd
www.lifecoachingacademy.com

The Coaches Training Institute
www.thecoaches.com

The Oxford School of Coaching and Mentoring
www.oscm.co.uk

The School of Coaching
www.theschoolofcoaching.com

These are just a few of the organisations offering training courses. For a fuller list see the ICF website: www.coachfederation.org/training/organizations.htm

Other resources

Doctor Healer Network
Contact Michael Dibdin
Tel: +44 (0)208 800 3569 (UK)

Eurocoach List
E-group network of coaches
www.ukcoachlist.com

International Stress Management Association
www.isma.org.uk

The Coaching and Mentoring Network
www.coachingnetwork.org.uk

Coach directory

A directory of career, corporate and personal coaches and their specialities. Coaches appear in alphabetical order. The following abbreviations denote certification levels awarded by the International Coach Federation:
PCC = Professional Certified Coach
MCC = Master Certified Coach.
Before calling coaches overseas, you are recommended to email first and check their time zone.

Shirley Anderson
MS CMC MCC
Coach Miami, Inc.
Helping you prioritise and reach your life goals and dreams.
Tel: 1-605-329-2622 (USA)
shirley@coachmiami.com
www.coachmiami.com

Ronald F Arndt
DDS MBA MAGD
The Dental Coach
Tel: 1-440-748-6161 (USA)
DrRon@DrArndt.com
www.DrArndt.com

Ginny Baillie
Baillie and Friends (B&F) *The coaching company for self-employed and business owners who want to stretch beyond the possible and create some extraordinary results.*
A company evolves on the characteristics of its major player - that's YOU.
Tel: +44 (0)187 385 7344
ginny@bandf.org
www.bandf.org

Bernadette Baker
Stress Management Consultant,
Business Coach and Author.
Empowering minds to better times.
Tel: +44 (0)151 480 6445
info@lifecoacher.com
www.lifecoacher.com

Linda Bark
RN PhD
Helping people make health changes.
Founder/Director of Whole Health Coaching Institute - Continuing education for professionals. Coaching from a body/mind/spirit perspective.
Tel: 1-510-864-1975 (USA)
lbark7777@aol.com
www.wholehealthcoaching.com

Laura Berman-Fortgang
Intercoach: The Coaching Company
Life Strategies - Business Results - Focus To Achieve
Tel: 1-973-857-8180 (USA)
lbf@intercoach.com
www.intercoach.com

Gabrielle Blackman-Sheppard
FMUKCLC
The woman coach passionate about coaching men. Coaching towards ManPower through gut, heart and soul.
Tel: +44 (0)870 241 4427
gabrielle@direktion-coaching.com
www.direktion-coaching.com

Nancy Boyd
BSc Certified Bach Flower Essence Therapist
Personal and professional coach specialising in cultural creatives, reorientating Indigo families around a soul-based operating system, and group coach training.
Tel: 1- 888-833-1725 voicemail (USA)
1- 914-944-0124 direct/fax (USA)
brightwings@att.net or
nancy@daytoppers.com
www.daytoppers.com and
www.findacoach.com/coach/brightwings.ci

Jane Brendgen
Life coach specialising in enhancing performance and well-being. Areas of focus include stress management and self-esteem issues.
Tel: +44 (0)162 889 8019
jbrendgen@onetel.net.uk
www.stressence.co.uk

Kimberly Bryant
PCC Certified Coach U graduate
Business and personal coach specialising in effective communication, life and career transitions, aging issues and self-employed business success.
Tel: 1-719-256-4786 (USA)
timecoach@kimberlybryant.com
www.kimberlybryant.com

Mani Bush
AAdip Dip IATE ITEC LCA
Life coach - developing environments to enhance emotional intelligence, proactivity and success, specialising in the fields of education, healthcare and empowerment through creativity.
Tel: +44 (0)179 958 4727 / 123
manitara@globalnet.co.uk
www.lifecoachingforsuccess.com

Jenna Caplette
Inward journey coach
Nature coach specialising in developing and integrating lessons and metaphors from the natural world into our work, and our lives.
Tel: 1-406-920-2691 (USA)
jennac@in-tch.com
www.communityzero.com/inwardjourney

Dr Chris Carling
Personal and Business Coach, ICF accredited
Specialising in communication, better personal and professional relationships and helping achieve focus and clarity.
Tel: 44 (0)122 336 7271
chris@chriscoach.com
www.chriscoach.com

Alicia Carter
CMT LCE
Health coach specialising in chronic and life-altering illness, as well as health passages such as menopause.
Tel: 1-510-841-0497 (USA)
ChrysalisHC@aol.com

Michele Lisenbury Christensen
PCC, certified mentor coach
Success coach who collaborates with clients to create spiritual bliss, financial freedom and career satisfaction.
Tel: 1-206-729-8497 (USA)
michele@successmadefun.com
www.successmadefun.com and
www.theevolutiongroup.com

Dr Margaret Collins
Life and business coach who works with women who want to make a difference, to become more through achieving their dreams.
Tel: +44 (0)118 962 2868
coaching@thegrowthzone.com
www.thegrowthzone.com

Rachelle Disbennett-Lee
MS MCC
Business and personal coach supporting professionals in being more productive and profitable while staying sane and balanced.
Tel: 1-303-617-6196 (USA)
rachelle@coachlee.com
www.365daysofcoaching.com

Alan Dobzinski
Executive coach and professional speaker
Executive coach providing business solutions and ideas with specialisation in leadership and accountability.
Tel: 1-410-296-6200 Extension 18 (USA)
AlanD@mksh.com
www.mksh.com

Susan Dunn
MA
Personal, career, emotional intelligence, and executive coaching.
Tel: 1-210-496-0678 (USA)
sdunn@susandunn.cc
www.susandunn.cc

Barbara Edwards BA(Oxon) DMS
Barbara Edwards Associates
Personal and business coach specialising in wellbeing, social relationships and dealing with difficult people.
Tel: +44 (0)148 383 2250
becoach@ntlworld.com
www.barbaraedwards.co.uk

Elizabeth Ferguson MCC
One of the first European coaches awarded independent accreditation by the ICF and founder of Duncan MacQuarrie Associates Ltd. Bringing coaching and consulting to organisations wanting to be their best.
Tel: +44 (0)870 751 8822
info@DuncanMacQuarrie.com
www.DuncanMacQuarrie.com

Mark Forster
Life coach, author and speaker specialising in time management and personal organisation.
Tel: +44 (0)140 324 0016
mf@markforster.net
www.markforster.net

Nancy Gambrell
BA
coachable2@aol.com

Gabriella Goddard MICF MCIM
Business and personal coach for people who want to stretch the boundaries of possibility.
Tel: +44 (0)207 394 8503
ggoddard@claravia.com
www.claravia.com

Dr Anne D Gooding PhD/DSW CSW
Coaching for the healthcare professional. Expertise in coaching healthcare professionals in personal, life, business and career transitions, goal setting and problem solving.
Tel: 1-914-997-2215 (USA)
coaching@adgsms.com
www.ADGSMS.COM

Suzy Greaves
CoachU Graduate
Big Leap one-to-one health coaching coaches clients to create a truly healthy life where clients look after themselves at such a high level that life feels positively luxurious.
Tel: +44 (0)208 980 4435
suzy@thebig-leap.com
www.thebig-leap.com

Soleira Green
Quantum coach specialising in personal and organisational strategic visioning.
Tel: +44 (0)138 073 9893
Soleira@SOULutions.co.uk
www.CorporateSOULutions.com and www.ExecuVision.net

Bob Griffiths ACA
Business and life coach specialising in helping professionals build the life they want rather than the life they have got.
Tel: +44 (0)207 787 8599
coach@willow.demon.co.uk
www.coachmaster.co.uk/coachmaster/index.html

Coen de Groot
I specialise in bringing coaches together, creating places where sparks fly.
Tel: +44 (0)117 955 0062
coen@coachcoen.com
www.CoachCoen.com

Ruth Hadikin
BSc(Hons) CoachU Graduate Cert Ed ADM RM RN
Business and life coach specialising in emotional intelligence (EQ), stress management and personal, professional and organisational development. International coaching by phone and email. Know yourSelf-Love yourSelf-Be yourSelf.
Tel: +44 (0)170 489 6039
ruth@dreamcoach.co.uk
www.dreamcoach.co.uk

Gina Harris
Access coaching, life and business coaching.
Tel: +44 (0)133 535 0540
info@accesscoaching.co.uk
www.accesscoaching.co.uk

Kirsten Hearn
NLP master practitioner,
NLP certified coach (ITS),
MA (RCA)
Empowerment coach and change consultant assisting people to become leaders in and of their lives, especially those from disadvantaged communities.
Tel: +44 (0)207 281 0852
kirsten@flotowers.freeserve.co.uk
www.wholeworlddesign.co.uk

Frances (Fran) Henry RDH
Personal and business coach working with people and businesses to create a happy, healthy and wealthy lifestyle.
Tel: 1-386-753-0323 (USA)
fdhcoach@yahoo.com
www.franhenry.com

Laura Hess
SPARCK International: Success - Personal power - Answers - Results - Choice - Knowledge.
Imagine the possibilities.
Tel: 1-702-252-4551 (USA)
laura@sparckint.com
www.sparckint.com

Steven Hunt
RGN BSc DHyp
Corporate development coach specialising in healthcare and work related stress management. Offers dynamic on-site workshops with support coaching.
Tel: +44 (0)175 286 3066
or +44 (0)776 256 5429
mind.tec@virgin.net
www.mind-tec.com

Judith Ideker
MA Psychology
20 years of business experience with healthcare professionals. Business and life coach specialising in professional women who want their lives to be the best expression of themselves.
Tel: 1-865- 693-5722 (USA)
judith@idekercoaching.com
www.idekercoaching.com

Gerard Jakimavicius BPharm CoachU Graduate
Business and life coach working with people who want special results and lots of happiness - achieved with heaps of fun and creativity!
Tel: +44 (0)19 498 1125
gerard@life-coach-associates.com
www.life-coach-associates.com

Sue Jamieson
Personal and business life coach, member of the International Coach Federation.
Jamiesonsue@hotmail.com
www.DiscoverYourBest.com

Maya Jordan
Coaching and programmes for realizing human potential.
Tel: 1-831-335-3477 (USA)
maya@aimingforexcellence.com
www.aimingforexcellence.com

Susan E. Kersley
MB BCh BA MEd
Enabling doctors to live the life they truly want.
Tel: +44 (0)1736 810 079
susan@youcanchangeyourlife.co.uk
www.thedoctorscoach.co.uk

Dianna Keel
Futurevisions: creating sustainable results in growth and performance.
Tel: +44 (0)208 780 9240
dianna@FutureVisions.org
www.futurevisions.org

Guy Levine
Working with people to combine marketing, customer service and technology to build 'better' and more profitable business relationships.
Tel: +44 (0)870 787 4372
guy@levineit.com
www.levineit.com

Jenny Linton-Beresford
BA MEd MCIPD
Career and business coach specialising in helping professionals to find or create work that's true to them.
Tel: +44 (0)115 967 3169
mail@heartwork-coach.co.uk
www.heartwork-coach.co.uk

Sarah Litvinoff
Respected author of self-help books, who works with talented, intelligent people who want support to make changes in their lives.
Tel: 44 (0)207 729 3115
sarahl@dircon.co.uk

Arlene Mann
CoachU graduate and faculty member. Masters degree in consciousness international consulting and coaching.
Specialising in professional and personal development, Arlene is a business and life coach with the added edge of being an extraordinarily gifted intuititve.
Your uniqueness ~ is ~ your success.
Tel: 1-603-883-9320 (USA)
Arlene@ArleneMann.com
www.ArleneMann.com

Linda Markley
BA
Personal and business coach specialising in sensitive people and those who want to live deeper, more fulfilled lives.
Tel: +44 (0)845 123 5109
(local rate calls in UK)
linda@clovercoaching.com
www.clovercoaching.com

Carolyn Matheson BSc(Hons) MCC
Business coach who has pioneered an innovative approach to coaching, combining high performance coaching with holistic approach to work/life balance.
Tel: +44 (0)208 269 0993
carolyn@fulcrum-hrm.co.uk
www.peopleworkbest.com

Jane MacAllister Dukes
TNM coaching UK
Quantum coach working in the moment and energetically with people who are open to exploration and discovery, where together we can create what alone we can only dream.
Tel: +44 (0)179 722 9537
jane@tnmcoaching.com
www.tnmcoaching.com

George Metcalfe
Tel: +44 (0)208 670 2122
GeorgeFMetcalfe@aol.com
www.georgemetcalfe.com

Nancy Morris
Nancy, CEO of Puddlejumping.com and Phoenix Coaching, works with people who are really ready to create an adventure from their relocation, in both their professional and personal lives.
Tel: +44 (0)283 025 6775
Nancy@puddlejumping.com
www.puddlejumping.com

John S Nagy
MSEM
Professional business and personal coach specialising in clarifying, strategising, planning and causing next-level activities without the usual associated hassles.
Tel: 1-813-949-0718 (USA)
NextLevel@coach.net
www.coach.net

Michael Neill
BFA certifed trainer of NLP
Certified trainer of Neuro-Linguistic Programming (NLP); has been coaching CEOs, writers, actors, and even royalty for the past 13 years.
Tel: 1-818-340-4464 (USA -Pacific time)
michael@successmadefun.com
www.successmadefun.com

Sarah Newton
Teen coach specialising in creating positive, rewarding and supportive partnerships between adults and teenagers.
Tel: +44 (0)870 751 8825
sarah@coaching4teens.com
www.coaching4teens.com

Muriel O'Driscoll
MA RM MTD Stress management dip, Dip psychosexual therapy
Coach/therapist specialising in stress management, work, financial, relationship and sexual problems.
'When you are stuck, I help you move forward.'
Tel: +44 (0)151 928 0596
muriel@uwrite.co.uk
www.murielodriscoll.co.uk

Karen Ormiston *Putting people first.*
We work with clients who are willing to invest in their most valuable asset - people. Individually and in groups.
Tel: +44 (0)161 374 5610
karen@resources4.co.uk
www.resources4.co.uk

Blaire Palmer
BA(Hons) Coach U Graduate
Executive, business and personal coach specialising in motivation and leadership, small business success and life purpose coaching.
Tel: +44 (0)208 574 2469
blaire@dreamcatcher-coaching.com
www.dreamcatcher-coaching.com

Jay Perry
Tel: 1-434- 245-7039 (USA)
JPcoach@aol.com
www.coachingcollective.com

Julie Plenty
Designer of self-coaching programmes personal and business coach specialising in creating self-coaching programmes on kickstarting self-esteem, goal setting and motivation.
Tel: +44 (0)845 122 0491
julie@kickstartyourselfesteem.com
www.kickstartyourselfesteem.com

Sue Pouppirt
PCC Professional Coach
Discover yourself and realize that out of that discovery is every answer you will ever need.
Tel: 1-970-224-9903 (USA)
sue@sensitivepeople.com
www.sensitivepeople.com

Susan E Race
PCC
Career and life coach specialising in compelling careers and relationships, job security for life, and building collaborative business organisations.
Tel: 1- 610- 695 -0464 (USA)
susanrace@erols.com
www.personalgrowthsystems.com

Lorna M S Ramsay
MA(Hons) Dip Ed
Graduate of CoachU, Assoc. Graduate School of Coaching, ICF Scottish Chapter Host. Director: The Kelvin Consultants Ltd. Personal achievement and business coach.
Tel: +44 (0)147 556 0007
thecoach@kelvin.org
www.kelvin.org

Naomi Rose
MA Book developer
Creator of Writing From the Deeper Self (WFDS). Using the WFDS approach, I help you bring the beauty that is you into written form and into the world.
Tel: 1-510-465-3935 (USA)
naomierose@yahoo.com
www.essentialwriting.com

Anna Rushton
Creative life strategist.
Tel: +44 (0)127 358 8817
anna@creativecatalyst.co.uk
www.creativecatalyst.co.uk

Aboodi Shabi
ICF Associate Certified Coach, CoachU Graduate
Deep conversations to explore your life fully and give you more freedom and meaning from life.
Tel: +44 (0)1273 719683
coach@aboodi.net
www.freedomconversations.com

Jilly Shaul
PCC CUCG
Certified teleclass leader and jump start coach. 'Life is either a daring adventure or nothing' (Helen Keller).
Tel: +44 (0)208 275 0072 (Practice)
+44 (0)208 449 3154 (House/Fax)
lifematters@btinternet.com
www.lifematters.co.uk

Dr John Stephenson
An experienced, certified coach specialising in business development for professionals, and coaching for personal/professional excellence.
Tel: 1-410-604-3899 (USA)
drjohn@coachingdoc.com
www.coachingdoc.com

Annabel Sutton
BA ACC
Life coach specialising in new business start-ups, decluttering your life, work/life balance, time management and confidence building.
Tel: +44 (0)162 558 4518
annabel@life-designs.co.uk

Lisbeth Tanz-Harrison MBA MICF
Personal and professional coach. LifeDance - A coaching practice.
Tel: 1-636-461-1690 (USA)
Lis@lifedance.net
www.lifedance.net

Zoran Todorovich
MCC
Personal and business coach specialising in attraction, spiritual, emotional and quantum intelligence coaching.
Tel: +46-708-860778
zoran@tnmcoaching.com
www.tnmcoaching.com

Natali Tremblay
Life purpose coach
Intuitive coach, focusing on personal life purpose quest.
Tel: 1-860-887-1877 (USA)
nat@TheIntuitive.com
www.TheIntuitive.com

Sandy Tremp
Life coach
Life changes counselling and coaching. Coaching woman to woman through life's changes. Discover yourself... love yourself... be the magnificent you.
Tel: 1- 602-439-1177 (USA)
lifechanges@qwest.net
www.lifechangescoach.com

Scott M Tremp
MC Counsellor, Life Coach
Life changes counselling and coaching. Coaching individuals and families through life's changes. Specialising in personal growth, parenting and men's self-awareness.
Tel: 1- 602-439-1177 (USA)
lifechanges@qwest.net
www.lifechangescoach.com and
www.lifechangescounseling.com

Rachel Turner
BA PCC
My clients are freethinkers who want to create the business of their dreams.
Tel: +44 (0)144 440 0034
rachel@kaizencoaching.com
www.kaizencoaching.com

Amechi Udo
MA MCIPD Perf. Coaching Dip [Bus] CNLP
Personally create your career of choice by working with an experienced career coach focused on helping you maximise your talents.
Tel: +44 (0)208 959 0566
+44 (0)845 125 7359 (local rate calls in UK)
amechi@pc4yc.co.uk
www.pc4yc.co.uk

Lisa Wynn
MCSP SRP MICF SAC Dip (Nutrition)
Chartered physiotherapist, nutritionist and life and business coach.
Success from within.
Tel: +44 (0)132 343 9166
lisa@perfectlifecompany.com
www.perfectlifecompany.com

Index

A

B

C

J

K

L

M

N

O

P

Q

R

S

T